The Art and Art Therapy of Papermaking

*The Art and Art Therapy of Paperm*aking: *Material, Methods, and Applications* provides a comprehensive collection about the contemporary practices, media, and value of hand papermaking as social engagement, art therapy, and personal voice.

Divided into three parts that highlight each of these areas, contributors explore topics such as advocacy, work with survivors, community outreach, medical challenges, and how papermaking can empower creative expression, stories of change, recovery, and reclamation to address trauma, grief and loss, social action, and life experiences. Previous books have covered hand papermaking or art therapy media as stand-alone subjects; this text is the first of its kind that unites and describes the convergence of papermaking in all these forms.

Art therapists, art educators, and artists will find this book essential to their education about how papermaking can be a powerful process to make meaning for the self, groups, and community.

Drew Luan Matott is a Master Papermaker and Founder and Director of the Peace Paper Project with expertise in using papermaking as a form of social engagement and community activism.

Gretchen M. Miller is a Registered Board Certified Art Therapist and Advanced Certified Trauma Practitioner.

"In *The Art and Art Therapy of Papermaking: Material, Methods, and Applications*, editors Drew Luan Matott and Gretchen M. Miller have gathered an important series of essays by practitioners who have seen, again and again, how therapeutic the craft can be. This book is essential for anyone who cares about the craft of papermaking, and its ability to help nurture and heal."

Tim Barrett, *director emeritus, University of Iowa Center for the Book*

"This wonderful book is what happens when artists and art therapists get together to rediscover an age-old yet uncommon material. Every aspect of papermaking is described: from how to approach this fascinating medium and invite participants to explore its alchemical potential, to the practical details and endless therapeutic adaptations that can be made. But it doesn't stop there: More than a book on papermaking, it offers a soul-stirring testimony to the work of reclamation – as people courageously free the fibers of their military uniforms, baby blankets, public records, t-shirts, love and hate letters, and more – to be pulped, recast, and transformed with radical insights that inspire far-reaching transformations in their lives."

Lynn Kapitan, Ph.D., ATR-BC, HLM, *professor emeritus of graduate and doctoral art therapy and author,* Introduction to Art Therapy Research

"The Art & Art Therapy of Papermaking is an accessible guide to transforming meaningful materials and experiences into sheets of paper and works of art. An insightful book filled with examples of healing through the papermaking process – the first of its kind!"

Helen Hiebert, *author,* The Papermaker's Companion, *artist, and educator*

"Serendipity often led contributors to this book to papermaking. Fortunately, readers can engage with papermaking more intentionally and knowledgeably with Matott and Miller's *The Art and Art Therapy of Papermaking* as their guide. Teachers, art activists, art therapists, students, and artists of all experience levels will find practical and inspirational material here. The book is replete with examples, instructions, and resources that are relatable and accessible. The authors have made papermaking, often perceived as too complicated for novice users, approachable by all. Highly Recommended!"

Lisa D. Hinz, Ph.D., ATR-BC *author,* Expressive Therapies Continuum A Framework for Using Art in Therapy

The Art and Art Therapy of Papermaking

Material, Methods, and Applications

Edited by

Drew Luan Matott
Gretchen M. Miller

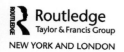

Routledge
Taylor & Francis Group

NEW YORK AND LONDON

Designed cover image: © Getty

First published 2024
by Routledge
605 Third Avenue, New York, NY 10158

and by Routledge
4 Park Square, Milton Park, Abingdon, Oxon, OX14 4RN

Routledge is an imprint of the Taylor & Francis Group, an informa business

Library of Congress Cataloging-in-Publication Data
Names: Matott, Drew Luan, editor. | Miller, Gretchen M., editor.
Title: The art and art therapy of papermaking : material, methods, and applications / edited by Drew Luan Matott, Gretchen M. Miller.
Description: New York, NY : Routledge, 2024. | Includes bibliographical references and index. | Identifiers: LCCN 2023009850 (print) | LCCN 2023009851 (ebook) | ISBN 9781032106243 (hardback) | ISBN 9781032106236 (paperback) | ISBN 9781003216261 (ebook)
Subjects: LCSH: Papermaking--Therapeutic use. | Art therapy--Methodology.
Classification: LCC RC489.A7 A738 2024 (print) | LCC RC489.A7 (ebook) | DDC 616.89/1656--dc23/eng/20230503
LC record available at https://lccn.loc.gov/2023009850
LC ebook record available at https://lccn.loc.gov/2023009851

ISBN: 9781032106243 (hbk)
ISBN: 9781032106236 (pbk)
ISBN: 9781003216261 (ebk)

DOI: 10.4324/9781003216261

Typeset in Times New Roman
by KnowledgeWorks Global Ltd.

For the activists, collaborators, survivors, and those who have stepped out of their comfort zones to blend disciplines and break new ground to support individuals and communities

Contents

Figures and Tables

Figures

Tables

About the Editors

Drew Luan Matott, M.F.A. (https://orcid.org/0000-0001-7691-1159) is a Master Papermaker with expertise in using traditional papermaking as a form of global social engagement and community activism. He received his M.F.A. in book and paper arts from Columbia College-Chicago and his B.F.A. in printmaking from Buffalo State College. Drew has taught and exhibited internationally and completed numerous artist residencies. He cofounded the Green Door Studio (2002), the Combat Paper Project (2007), Peace Paper Project (2011), Veteran Paper Workshop (2011), and St. Pauli Paper (2016). Drew lives in Hamburg, Germany. where he divides his time between teaching for the Volkshochschule, completing studio work, and designing new papermaking endeavors for Peace Paper Project. In 2019 he was the recipient of the American Art Therapy Association's Rudolph Arnheim Award, designated for a non-member of the Association whose contributions have significantly impacted the art therapy profession. Learn more about Drew's work at drewmatott.com.

Gretchen M. Miller, M.A., A.T.R.-B.C., A.T.C.P. (https://orcid.org/0000-0003-4165-517X) is a Registered Board Certified Art Therapist and Advanced Certified Trauma Practitioner in Northeast Ohio, United States. Over the last 20 years, her art therapy work has included serving youth and adults impacted by trauma and loss. Gretchen is an art therapy educator, regional, national, and international speaker, author, supervisor, and community organizer. Since 2011, Gretchen has served as a co-director of the Peace Paper Project. In collaboration with Drew Matott, she has helped develop Peace Paper Project coursework and workshops, including consultation to art therapists and art therapy students seeking to learn more about the therapeutic qualities of papermaking as a form of trauma intervention and recovery. Learn more about Gretchen's work at gretchen-miller.com.

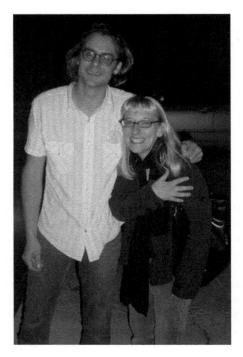

Figure 0.1 Drew and Gretchen's first meeting at The Morgan Paper Conservatory in Cleveland, Ohio, 2009.

Contributors

Courtney Bowles is an artist, educator, and community organizer. Her projects combine coordinating strategies and urgently needed services with collaborative, poetic, and performative actions that connect diverse and often antagonistic actors. She currently co-directs the People's Paper Co-op and the Reentry Think Tank in Philadelphia, Pennsylvania.

Amy Bucciarelli, M.S., A.T.R.-B.C., L.M.H.C., N.C.C. (https://orcid.org/0000-0003-4305-6031) is a Board Certified Art Therapist and Licensed Mental Health Counselor in Florida, United States. She owns Coastal Blossom Counseling & Art Therapy, specializing in medical art therapy, trauma, and loss. Amy taught graduate-level art therapy and arts in medicine for over a decade. She began papermaking in 2012, thanks to Peace Paper Project.

Genevieve S. Camp, M.A., L.M.H.C., A.T.R.-B.C., C.E.D.S. (https://orcid.org0000-0003-2663-5912) is a Licensed Mental Health Counselor, Registered Board Certified Art Therapist, and Certified Eating Disorder Specialist in private practice in Florida, United States. With specialized training in Internal Family Systems (I.F.S.) and Eye Movement Desensitization and Reprocessing(E.M.D.R.) therapies, Genevieve's work focuses on treating the intersection of developmental/relational trauma and eating disorders.

Jennifer L. Davis (http://www.orcid.org/0000-0001-9499-1826) holds a Master's degree in education and, at the time of publication, is working on a Master's degree in Marriage and Family Therapy. She provides therapy to individuals, couples, and families. In addition, Jennifer conducts papermaking workshops and other therapeutic art classes for groups and communities in Kansas, United States.

Raoul Deal, M.V.A., B.F.A. (http://www.orcid.org/0000-0003-4894-1654) received his M.V.A. from the Universidad Nacional Autónoma de México in painting and is the founding Coordinator of the Community Arts B.A. Program at the University of Wisconsin-Milwaukee (U.W.M.), United States. A Senior Lecturer in the Peck School of the Arts, Raoul has served as Artist-in-Residence for U.W.M.'s Cultures and Communities Program since 2002.

Janice M. Havlena, B.F.A., M.A., A.T.R.-B.C.-Retired (https://orcid. org/0000-0003-3763-4202) received her M.A. in art therapy from the University of New Mexico and her B.F.A. from Wayne State University, Detroit, United States. Her work has included clinical art therapy, academic teaching, research in epilepsy, art therapy, and community art. Janice has collaborated with Peace Paper Project since 2012.

Meadow Jones, Ph.D. completed her M.L.I.S. and Ph.D. at the University of Illinois Urbana-Champaign, United States. Her dissertation, *Archiving the Trauma Diaspora*, concerned the use of art practices in the redress of trauma. She facilitates trauma-responsive writing workshops and training. Dr. Jones is currently a student at the Maitreya Buddhist Seminary.

Steven Kostell, M.F.A. (http://www.orcid.org/0000-0002-5940-1496) is a visual artist and designer whose work is grounded in material-based production, incorporating waste streams and natural materials through hand papermaking. He serves as Assistant Professor at The University of Vermont where he leads the U.V.M. Biofiber Lab, focusing on circular design systems through regenerative material exploration.

Tom Lascell is a paper and book artist living in northern New York. He has worked with both the Combat Paper Project and the Peace Paper Project. His series of pulp paper masks have traveled with the Combat Paper Project, and they have been exhibited in the United Kingdom and several venues within the United States.

Nathan Lewis is an artist, writer, activist, and arborist living near Ithaca, New York. In addition, he is an U.S. army veteran who served in Iraq. Nathan's work has been shown across the country and is in many rare book collections. He has facilitated veteran workshops with the Combat Paper Project, Frontline Arts, Community Building Art Works, and Peace Paper Project.

Annie McFarland, Ph.D., A.T.R.-B.C., (http://www.orcid.org/0000-0001-6064-5060) is an art therapist, educator. She works as an Assistant Professor of Art Therapy at West Virginia University. Her current research includes trauma recovery through art therapy and the I.T.R. method. Dr. McFarland has clinical experience working in inpatient psychiatric centers, with palliative care, and with military populations.

Meredith Lin McMackin, M.F.A., M.S., Ph.D., L.M.H.C., A.T.R (https:// orcid.org/0000-0002-0691-3607) received an M.F.A. in Studio Art, an M.S. in Art Therapy, and a Ph.D. in Art Education from Florida State University. While attending Florida State, she researched the therapeutic process of hand papermaking with student veterans. Dr. McMackin works as an Art Therapist and Licensed Mental Health Counselor in Vancouver, Washington, United States.

Rachel Mims, M.S., A.T.R.-B.C., L.P.C.-A.T. (https://orcid.org/0000-0003-0199-8098) is a Board Certified Art Therapist and U.S. army veteran. She has a passion for helping women, veterans, and queer folks recover from trauma. Rachel has worked in a variety of settings including community mental health, non-profits, higher education, private practice, and telehealth.

Amy Koski Richard, M.F.A. (https://orcid.org/0000-0003-0698-5552) received her M.F.A. in Book Arts from the University of Iowa, Center for the Book, and B.F.A. in Studio Art from Lamar University, United States. A visual artist and writer, Amy's papermaking practice serves as a conduit to the natural environment as well as spiritual and healing connections that she shares with others.

John Risseeuw, M.F.A. received his M.F.A. in Printmaking from the University of Wisconsin-Madison. An Emeritus Professor at Arizona State University (A.S.U.), he taught printmaking, bookmaking, and papermaking for over 40 years. He also established A.S.U.'s book arts press Pyracantha Press. John's own press, Cabbagehead Press was founded in 1972; it is in Tempe, Arizona, United States.

Erin Mooney-Simkus, L.C.P.C., A.T.R.-B.C. is a Licensed Clinical Professional Counselor and Board Certified Art Therapist. Her clinical work includes working with adults managing anxiety, trauma, and loss. She also specializes in L.G.B.T.Q.A. support. Erin is a professor, supervisor, and the founder of Create Balance Counseling, an art therapy practice in Illinois, United States.

Mark Strandquist is Co-director of People's Paper Co-op and Performing Statistics. He has spent years using art to help amplify, celebrate, and power social justice movements. Blending public art, cultural organizing, and interactive technology, his work operates at a monumental scale reaching hundreds of thousands of viewers without compromising a deeply collaborative practice.

Yaslin M. Torres-Peña serves as Student Engagement Liaison for Washington State University's Undocumented Initiatives program in Pullman, Washington, United States.

Denise R. Wolf, A.T.C.S., L.P.C., L.P.A.T. (https://orcid.org/0000-0002-7479-4662) is an artist and art therapist. She is an Associate Clinical Professor at Drexel University and the owner and practitioner/therapist of Mangata Services. Denise believes a neurological understanding of trauma eliminates judgment and creates opportunities for community action care through therapeutic arts processes.

Eli Wright enlisted as a U.S. army medic after September 11, 2001. Upon returning home from Iraq in 2004, he began organizing with other veterans to speak out about their military experiences through activism and the arts. Since 2007, Eli has practiced the craft of making handmade paper from military uniforms with veterans from across the country.

Acknowledgments

The topic of this book is the art and art therapy of papermaking, but its foundation is deeply grounded in collaboration and community.

We are truly grateful to the 20 authors who contributed their experiences, knowledge, time, and attention to the development of this seminal book and its chapters. Thank you, John, Raoul, Steve, Meadow, Amy B., Genevieve, Amy R., Janice, Meredith, Mark, Courtney, Jenny, Tom, Nathan, Annie, Rachel, Erin, Yaslin, Denise, and Eli. We also extend our sincere appreciation to the many contributors and participants who generously provided permission to share their art, creative work, and stories throughout the three parts of this book. We thank and recognize Casey Boone, Emma Krueger, Dr. Sheila Lorenzo de la Peña, Lee McDonald, and Patrick Sargent for their inspiring interview participation as part of Chapter 8. A special thank you to artist, psychiatrist, and activist Dr. Eric Avery for contributing the Foreword for this book.

Individuals who helped review content and provided feedback at different stages of the book's development included: Tim Barrett, Dr. David Gussak, Christie Knoll, Lynne Matott, Nannie Mead, Dr. Jordan Potash, Patrick Sargent, and Dr. Mary Jo Zygmond. Your collective reviews and contributions helped strengthen this book from its conception to the final draft. Thank you! We also express much thanks to Routledge's editor and production teams, including Commissioning Editor Amanda Devine and Editorial Assistants Kayta Porter and Priya Sharma for their encouragement and assistance throughout this process.

Additionally, we want to thank the numerous individuals, communities, and groups that have supported the work and mission of the Peace Paper Project, papermaking as social engagement, and papermaking as art therapy. This network includes but is not limited to, college campuses, university and academic programs, faculty, students, and workshop participants, as well as medical, mental health, cultural, and membership organizations across the U.S. and internationally.

On a personal note: *from Drew*: thank you to my papermaking professors Melissa Jay Craig, Paul D. Martin, Andrea Peterson, Masha Ryskin, Peter Sowiski, and Marylin Sward, who gave me solid technical training while encouraging me to push the boundaries of papermaking as an art form. *From Gretchen*: an expression of thanks to art therapy mentors and colleagues Dr. Sister Kathleen Burke, Dr. Michael Franklin, Dr. Lani Gerity Glanville, Dr. Lynn Kapitan, and Drs. Bruce and Cathy Moon. Your teachings, writings, and work has helped inform and inspire my creative practice and unique attention to the power of unconventional media, processes, and materials as an artist and art therapist.

Last, but certainly not least, we acknowledge our partners, Jana Schumacher and Kevin King with our deepest gratitude, as well as a heartfelt thanks to our family and friends for their unconditional support and love.

Drew Luan Matott and Gretchen M. Miller

Foreword

A lifelong printmaking art practice helped me cope with a traumatic childhood, my medical education, and to survive as the medical director in 1981 of a large feeding program in a refugee camp in Somalia. Then, in 1996, art saved my life when I became the AIDS psychiatrist at The University of Texas Medical Branch (U.T.M.B.) at Galveston. Part of my clinical time was protected by the Institute for Medical Humanities to make art that reflected what I did as an AIDS psychiatrist. I made many prints about HIV/AIDS and developed art actions that worked in the liminal space between art and medicine. Besides cutting templates to make my prints, I had begun making paper from hospital sheets and surgical towels to add content to my prints.

In 2006, I first worked with Drew Matott when he was an M.F.A. student at Columbia Center for Book Arts and Paper and I was a visiting artist/printmaker. For our project, I brought sheets of paper I had made from my worn-out Perry Ellis cotton workshirts. After cutting up the soft old shirts by the designer who had died of AIDS, I left bits of the shirt fragments in the paper pulp which showed in the finished paper. Drew helped letterpress print a folio on this paper, with an introduction and a set of photo engraving prints made from woodcut portraits of my patients. The portraits were made in woodcut frames about HIV risk, abuse, and trauma.

A year later, we worked together a second time on a World AIDS Day project at Boston University (B.U.). In a public art action in the student union, Drew assisted B.U. students and faculty in sheet formation and screen printing over beaten pulp text onto the wet sheets of paper that read "Everyone Can Be A Leader On HIV/AIDS."

Drew's papermaking project as social engagement continued in Vermont at the Green Door Studio. After meeting Drew Cameron in 2007, a veteran who had recently returned from Iraq, they began working with other veterans returning home from war to make paper from their uniforms. The paper was used by the veterans for making art or for writing about their experiences. This became the Combat Paper Project. When Drew Matott began working with Gretchen Miller, a very experienced art therapist, their synergy led to the founding of the Peace Paper Project. This global project expanded the use of papermaking as a form of trauma intervention and recovery.

When neuroarthistorians study how art and art therapy reflected advances in the neuroscience of healing, they will find important evidence in this remarkable book. Neuroarthistory looks at creative productions by artists in the light of emerging neuroscience. Historically, sometimes artists and creatives discover something that works for them visually before neuroscience can explain it (Onians, 2008). My prints and later papermaking, especially in Somalia and in my HIV/AIDS clinical work, helped me process my experience of trauma. Drew and Gretchen do this with their work. Neuroscience is trying to understand how healing is facilitated by art-making (Van der Kolk, 2014). What does papermaking with lived cloth ("intentional fibers") add to this process of recovery and growth?

Understanding how to put the broken mind back together again is a goal of psychological and psychiatric therapy. How this works is a frontier of neuroscience. Trauma is common in those we try to help and teach. Severe traumas (verbal, emotional, physical, and sexual) can fragment the mind and break connections with the body. The word memory system can go "offline," resulting in traumatic memories being stored in emotional and body parts of the brain. Intergenerational transmission of trauma can occur without words about the trauma ever having been spoken. Because of this, words can only go so far in understanding and helping recover from trauma. Art often emerges from these dark places of suffering, almost like an M.R.I. from a broken soul. We learn to talk about and interpret these projections. We do this as teachers and therapists. How does art and paper made from cloth off our backs have the capacity to circumvent the trauma word storage and expression problem? How does the use of lived cloth bring the body/self into the moment so that it can speak for itself? When we work with this creative-making process, we look at and try to listen to what is being expressed.

An emerging question being asked in this book is how the use of papermaking with lived cloth facilitates healing. What does this papermaking add to the visual practice of helping the traumatized brain express itself or societies express communal grief? Drew and Gretchen help us understand this with this book. From their broad experiences in art, activism, and healing, they have gathered a group of artists, educators, art therapists, and community organizers to share their discoveries and pedagogies. Contributors write eloquently about their experiences and discoveries using handmade paper. The synergy of these practices and experiences in socially engaged art-making, papermaking and art therapy shows us a way to transform inner narratives that confine functioning in the world. We might not understand yet how this works, but *something* here is helping with trauma and recovery. I have made a lot of art in this space and have used it to help others understand and open their own narratives. The extensive bibliographies in this book are also a testament to how much we can learn from each other.

This book is structured in a way that moves the reader from the macro social self to the micro personal experiences of those who have used papermaking in their own journeys of growth and resilience. Readers will find much information on using papermaking in their practices. One can learn the basics of papermaking and sheet formation. I wish I had known how to make paper at the bedside of my patients on the AIDS wards. It is as simple as couching a small sheet of paper onto a sheet of plexiglass and leaving it on a windowsill to dry.

I will bookend what I write with experiences I have had with two contributors to the first and last sections of this remarkable book. I have worked with both. John Risseeuw describes his extraordinary project using clothing from landmine survivors in his art. He describes his personal journey as he discovered the power of papermaking with cloth that embodied lived trauma, horror, and survival. Besides raising money for survivors through sales, his artwork is fully represented in the Library of Congress. His prints and paper belong to the American people and will pass through time as a witness to the destruction caused by landmines in war and the resilience of the survivors. One day this will be part of neuroarthistory.

In 2013, I retired from my clinical practice to focus on my art practice and activism in New Hope, Pennsylvania. Not far from me, I was delighted to find that the Combat Paper Project had grown and was organized by David Keefe, an artist and veteran at the Printmaking Center of New Jersey. It is now called Frontline Arts. David invited me to several closed meetings to teach relief printmaking skills to veterans who were printing on their uniform-made paper. This is where I met Eli Wright. His contribution to this book, *Papermaking and the Process of Returning Home* is a model of what this book is about. How to heal the self, being present in the process of making paper from a uniform associated with horror and trauma. He can now eloquently describe his trauma and the process of recovering his narrative and voice using paper and printmaking.

I am honored to be asked by Drew and Gretchen to write a foreword to this remarkable and useful book. Much has happened since I first met Drew. At that time, I was trying to find a way to tell others about the connection between trauma and the HIV risk stories my patients were telling me. There was much suffering and dying in those days. My prints and papermaking helped me survive. It was my Art as Medicine. Now we can show you how to do it too.

Eric Avery M.D.
Emeritus Associate Professor
The Institute for Bioethics and Health Humanities
The University of Texas Medical Branch
Galveston, Texas
http://www.docart.com
http://www.ericaveryartist.com

References

Onians, J. (2008). *Neuroarthistory: From Aristotle and Pliny to Baxandall and Zeki.* Yale University Press

Van der Kolk, B. (2014). *The body keeps the score: Brain, mind and body in the healing of trauma.* Penguin Random House

Introduction

Drew Luan Matott and Gretchen M. Miller

Unexpected encounters can often introduce us to defining moments that inadvertently impact our lives, work, relationships, and sense of self. This is not uncommon in creative expression. Exposure to a new medium, a new technique, or a new idea can lead to valuable opportunities for self-discovery and ways of thinking (Botella et al., 2013). The process and act of hand papermaking, to which the forthcoming chapters are dedicated, introduces readers to how and why this medium has the profound capacity to create change. It inspires meaningful ways to serve as a form of advocacy, art therapy, and personal introspection.

Admittedly, we both have our own histories about the unknown potential of papermaking. Our first impressions and initial views lacked the knowledge about the transformative qualities inherent in the process. For example, cutting the rag of a meaningful article of clothing or cellulose material, pulping those fibers, pulling sheets, and then making art with the new paper can inspire a fresh beginning, a renewal, and activate life-altering narratives (Senchyne, 2020). Drew's first experience included reluctantly taking a required papermaking course during his undergraduate studies in printmaking. He found that he was influenced by the community spirit of the practice and the added layers of content when using rags of personal significance. This compelled him to keep learning about papermaking and ultimately determined his work as a master papermaker today. For Gretchen, making paper was primarily a fun craft activity she learned with recycled paper. In 2009 Gretchen first connected with Drew. As a result of this meeting, she was introduced to the tremendous potential the papermaking process could have as a therapeutic metaphor. This inspired and motivated her to learn how papermaking could be used in art therapy. A collaboration formed between Drew and Gretchen that brought together the enthusiasm and passion of their respective disciplines for the purpose of discovering ways to learn from each other and to connect with others regarding papermaking as forms of social action and art therapy. When Drew was co-directing the Combat Paper Project, he invited Gretchen to consult with the Project about art therapy (Ash, 2017; Gates, 2011; Vance, 2010). As Drew and Gretchen's partnership

DOI: 10.4324/9781003216261-1

grew, it included sharing papermaking applications and methods with the art therapy community through academic coursework and workshops. In 2011 increased attention to art therapy eventually broadened when they developed the Peace Paper Project, an international community–arts initiative that applies papermaking as trauma therapy, social engagement, and community activism through facilitating worldwide workshops. This partnership expanded as they worked on building a diverse papermaking network of practicing artists, art therapists, educators, community activists, university students, art studios, academic programs, and college campuses (Peace Paper Project, 2022). Many from this community have contributed to this book.

Contemporary Papermaking

This text highlights contemporary papermaking methods that have evolved from conventional practices that date to the second century B.C.E. (Hunter, 1974). Papermaking processes have advanced from laboriously pounding fibers by hand into pulp to create a single sheet of paper into mass paper production with industrialized manufacturing and equipment. The use and function of paper, even in its early beginnings, were deeply rooted in the ability to communicate, document, share information, narratives, and stories (Bloom, 2001).

Since the turn of the twenty-first century, papermakers have often used their artistic practice to empower social engagement, support community building, create collaboration, and promote awareness. Making paper by hand is an art form and an artistic process. The resulting artworks can chronicle the reconstruction and expression of personal and communal experiences, viewpoints of reflection, significant events, and encourage collaboration (Delamater, 2019). By using intentional fibers and processes loaded with history, content, and meaning, the papermaking process and accompanying artworks can become a platform for social action, community engagement, and culturally relevant issues (Barrett, 2018; Cochran & Potter, 2015).

In addition, art therapists are utilizing papermaking and its process as an intervention for art therapy. Influenced by its transmutation and sensory-based properties, art therapists use papermaking for promoting emotional expression, fostering self-awareness, or managing recovery, loss, and trauma (Matott & Miller, 2020). This becomes an important act of reclamation in the therapeutic frame for empowering self-definition, purpose, and coping. As a visible manifestation of resilience, reforming fibers into works of art invites opportunities for processing one's experience and story. Papermaking also creates opportunities to engage in and inform creative, relational dialogues, a critical therapeutic element of media and material use in art therapy (Dean, 2014). Papermaking practices introduce a refreshing shift from common and conventional art therapy applications, structures, and traditional art media historically used or taught in the field (Leone, 2020; Moon, 2010).

Papermaking Basics

Reading this book requires a working knowledge and general understanding of the basic tools, equipment, and processes of papermaking. The core material uniting all forms of papermaking is cellulose. One gathers cellulose and combines it with water. Sources of cellulose may be a raw plant, a letter or photograph, paper currency, a symbolic textile, or a significant article of clothing. Each fiber used has a unique story and narrative to tell, whether it is the geographic origin of the plant, the history of the landscape, or a personal connection to an experience or memory associated with the fiber.

Some papermaking basics we described in *The Routledge Companion to Health Humanities* are:

> The first steps of creating paper invites the maker into a safe framework to explore experiences, emotions, and sense of self through the process of cutting rag into small postage-stamp size pieces. This tearing, ripping, and pulling apart is a powerful creative act to honor, acknowledge, bring closure to, or explore experiences associated with these materials. Rag can come in the form of clothing, such as a military uniform, a hospital gown, a special T-shirt, or another emotionally significant garment. Cotton based textile items such as a family tablecloth, meaningful fabric, or paper-based material like photographs and letters can also be powerful to use in this process. There is something extraordinary that occurs when one begins breaking down the fiber. Participants may begin to share stories, memories, and important details connected to the material being altered. Common with other handmade art practices, reclaiming these fibers in this way helps translate the participant's memories, struggles, and feelings into a process of survival and restored life (Kapitan, 2011).
>
> This process of releasing and reforming is a fundamental step to help transform the papermaking experience as a means for personal expression, engagement, renewal, and as a representation of recovery and healing. The final step to "breaking rag" is to mix the pieces with water in a Hollander beater (if using fabric or cloth rag) or a household blender (if using paper rag), where the fiber material is beaten into a slurry pulp and ready to form into paper sheets with papermaking tools such as a mould and deckle. When the deckle is removed from the mould, the sheet is transferred onto an interface and then pressed to make the wet paper flat and strong. This process is known as couching. Techniques such as pulp printing, creative writing, bookmaking, collaging, and more can be used with the formed paper once dry.
>
> (Matott & Miller, 2020, p. 312)

Overview of This Book

The Art and Art Therapy of Papermaking: Material, Methods, and Applications provides a comprehensive collection of articles about the contemporary practices, media, and value of hand papermaking as social engagement, art therapy, and personal voice. While existing books focus separately on hand papermaking or materials in art therapy, this text is the first of its kind, uniting and describing the convergence of papermaking in all these forms. The contributing authors come from diverse backgrounds and experiences throughout the U.S. This includes service in the military, practicing studio artists and art facilitators, educators in academia, clinicians, researchers, and activists. The breadth of projects and narratives presented offer in-depth learning about how papermaking can be an art-based approach for social action, well-being, and personal growth. Furthermore, the content can be used to inform community-engaged initiatives, clinical work for art therapists, and creative expression.

Part I: Papermaking as Social Engagement

Part I is dedicated to the use of hand papermaking as a form of socially engaged art (S.E.A.). Chapter 1: *Making Paper Mean Something: Socially Engaged Art with Content-Specific Fibers* is written by John Risseeuw. The chapter describes the journey and evolution of the author's 40-year papermaking practice. During his journey, the author discovered how papermaking from significant fibers and articles of clothing may be applied beyond the aesthetic art product to embed handmade paper with unique, content-specific meaning. Chapter 2: *Pulp, Pull, Press, and Print: Engaging with Papermaking in Community Art Workshops*, authored by Raoul Deal, describes the papermaking experiences of community art students conducting intergenerational papermaking workshops. In partnership with youth groups, senior centers, and community organizations, student artists help create opportunities through papermaking for participants to manage aging, empower violence prevention in youth, and support grieving mothers of gun violence. Chapter 3: *Paper as Praxis*, by Steven Kostell and Meadow Jones, explores the transformative potential of hand papermaking as social engagement as it relates to building a community of practice. Through the lens of systems thinking, the authors discuss the intersections of modalities, stakeholders, materials, and processes as an activist approach toward social innovation.

Part II: Papermaking as Art Therapy

This section highlights papermaking as a form of art therapy and the therapeutic qualities inherent in its practice and process. Chapter 4: *Adaptations and Modifications for Therapeutic Hand Papermaking* is co-authored by Amy Bucciarelli, Genevieve S. Camp, and Amy Koski Richard. This chapter discusses unique adaptations and therapeutic aspects of hand papermaking methods that were applied to three distinct projects: a group process within an eating disorder treatment center; the development of a modular approach for bedside work with people hospitalized for medical conditions; and the integration of hand paper-making activities into a school curriculum for students with developmental disabilities. Chapter 5: *Papermaking Transformation in an Art Therapy Curriculum*, contributed by Janice M. Havlena, follows the journey of an undergraduate art therapy program and its community outreach across age, culture, and abilities. Along the way, students develop skills in papermaking and an appreciation for how this medium can give voice to youth, older adults, people living with epilepsy, and self-taught artists with disabilities. In addition, it also enhances the student's own art practice. Chapter 6: *Voices of the Bereaved: Papermaking for Processing Grief and Loss* written by Meredith Lin McMackin explores the therapeutic aspects of hand papermaking in working with individuals and groups experiencing grief and loss. Through interviews, individuals describe the process of transforming a cloth of significance related to their deceased loved one, and, with those fibers, creating a unique commemorative work of art. The author also shares her personal experience of loss and her engagement with papermaking.

Part III: Papermaking as Personal Voice

The book's final section includes a collection of ten first-person narratives about how papermaking has empowered personal stories of transformation. Chapter 7: *Papermaker Reflections: Stories of Change, Growth, and Creativity* includes: *The People's Paper Co-op* co-written by Courtney Bowles and Mark Strandquist; *A Personal Journey through Cancer, Papermaking, and Self-Transformation* authored by Jennifer L. Davis; *From Photographer to Papermaker and Book Artist: A Creative Odyssey* contributed by Tom Lascell; *Beating the War: Fighting Militarism through Papermaking* written by Nathan Lewis; *My Autoethnographic Research: Pulping My Late Father's T-shirts and Ties* authored by Annie McFarland; *Art Therapy Student to Art Therapist: Papermaking Lessons and Professional Practice* contributed by Rachel Mims; *When the Pulp Dries: Claiming the Self through Paper Exhibitions* written by Erin Mooney-Simkus; *Immigration, Advocacy, and Papermaking* contributed by Yaslin M. Torres-Peña; *Transformation in Papermaking: When Content Mirrors Process* authored by Denise R. Wolf, and the *Process of Returning Home* written by Eli Wright.

Conclusion and Back Matter

Chapter 8, *Future Thoughts and Directions* present outlooks and possibilities for the art and art therapy of papermaking as an enduring and emerging agent for social engagement, therapeutic intervention, and personal stories. The back matter of this book includes appendices that offer additional information and resources for learning more about and supporting the content presented in this book. A glossary of terms clarifies definitions and concepts mentioned throughout the book. Words and phrases included in the glossary are printed in bold when first referenced in each chapter.

Audience, Scope, and Uses of this Book

A range of audiences can benefit from reading this book. First, readers interested in new approaches related to socially engaged art, community outreach, and advocacy through creativity will find this book valuable to promote civic and psychosocial dialogue. Second, for art therapists this book offers theoretical considerations to incorporate therapeutic papermaking with numerous populations in different settings. Third, artists seeking to expand their creative practice, especially those interested in paper arts, printmaking, or book arts will be introduced to art-based ideas to consider. Academic programs, educators, and researchers can use this book to support their teaching, coursework, and inquiry. Those studying art therapy, fine art, craft, and health humanities can also learn from the book's topics and perspectives. Finally, experiences and reflections offered may be of special interest to anyone seeking connection to narratives and stories about art's ability to facilitate change, growth, and resiliency.

We close this introduction with a call to action. We invite you to consider how contemporary papermaking practices presented in this book could inspire, inform, and activate your own relational, professional, and creative contributions. Discover for yourself the potential of papermaking – as we once did.

References

Ash, J. (2017). The things paper carries: The combat paper project. *Art in Print, 6*(5), 11–15.

Barrett, T. D. (2018). *European hand papermaking: Traditions, tools, and techniques.* The Legacy Press.

Bloom, J. M. (2001). *Paper before print: The history and impact of paper in the Islamic world.* Yale University Press.

Botella, M., Glaveanu, V., Zenasni, F., Storme, M., Myszkowski, N., Wolff, M., & Lubart, T. (2013). How artists create: Creative process and multivariate factors, *Learning and Individual Differences, 26,* 161–170. https://doi.org/10.1016/j.lindif.2013.02.008.

Cochran, J., & Potter, M. H. (Eds.). (2015). *Social paper: Hand papermaking in the context of socially engaged art.* Columbia College Chicago Center for Book and Paper Arts.

Dean, M. L. (2014). *Using art media in psychotherapy.* Routledge.

Delamater, K. L. (2019). Historical, social, and artistic implications of collaboration in contemporary hand papermaking, *Hand Papermaking, 34* (1), 11–16.

Gates, B. (2011, June 7). *Combat papermakers Drew Cameron and Drew Matott: An interview in two voices.* Works and Conservation. https://www.conversations.org/story.php?sid=331.

Hunter, D. (1974). *Papermaking: The history and technique of an ancient craft.* Dover Publications.

Kapitan, L. (2011). Close to the heart: Art therapy's link to craft and art production. *Art Therapy: Journal of the American Art Therapy Association, 28*(3), 94–95. https://doi.org/10.1080/07421656.2011.601728.

Leone. L. (Ed.). (2020). *Craft in art therapy: Diverse approaches to the transformative power of craft materials and methods.* Routledge.

Matott, D. L., & Miller, G. M. (2020). Papermaking. In P. Crawford, B. J. Brown, & A. Charise (Eds). *The Routledge companion to health humanities* (pp. 311–316). Routledge.

Moon, C. H. (Ed.). (2010). *Materials & media in art therapy: Critical understandings of diverse artistic vocabularies.* Routledge.

Peace Paper Project. (2022). http://www.peacepaperprojectproject.org.

Senchyne, J. (2020). *The intimacy of paper in early and nineteenth century American literature.* University of Massachusetts Press.

Vance, R. (2010). *Rags to redemption: The Combat Paper Project.* HistoryNet. https://www.historynet.com/rags-to-redemption-the-combat-paper-project.htm.

Part I

Papermaking as Social Engagement

1 Making Paper Mean Something

Socially Engaged Art with Content-Specific Fibers

John Risseeuw

This chapter describes the journey and evolution of the author's 40-year paper-making practice. During his journey, the author discovered how papermaking from significant fibers and articles of clothing may be applied beyond the aesthetic art product to embed handmade paper with unique, content-specific meaning. This includes the author's individual account of a non-linear path toward the extraordinary potential and power of thoughtful papermaking. Examples particularly highlight the role of papermaking in social engagement and collaboration, as well as a creative, contemporary process for creating advocacy, education, and awareness for humanitarian aid.

Advocacy in art has been found in many artists' works from the social reform photography of Jacob Riis to Pablo Picasso's anti-war painting *Guernica*, and Barbara Kruger's postmodern feminist graphics. When Howard Zinn, an American historian and political scientist, stated, "In addition to creating works of art, the artist is also a citizen and a human being" (2007, p. 2), he was suggesting the artist may (and has a right to, perhaps even a responsibility to) examine world issues world through visual art and to advocate for understanding and change. When I began my journey as an artist, I could not have foreseen how much socially engaged concepts would eventually inform my work. Only with hindsight did I see this unfolding expansion of the medium.

Beginnings and Influences

In 1972 I first learned to make paper from cotton **rag** as a graduate art student at the University of Wisconsin-Madison (U.W.) (http://www.wisc.edu). At this time, the procedure was explained as a rather magical sequence of mechanical events without any reference to the actual physio-chemical processes:

- Cut up the cotton rag into pieces less than 1-inch square;
- Fill a **Valley Hollander beater** with water and turn it on;
- Slowly add the rag pieces until it "feels" full in the hand;

DOI: 10.4324/9781003216261-3

- Using a succession of weights on the lever arm, heavy to medium to light, let it beat until the rag has been reduced to thread and the thread has been reduced to fiber;
- Monitor and adjust beating pressure until you feel a slight "sliminess" to the **slurry**;
- Drain the beater and bring the **pulp** to a **vat** filled two-thirds with water;
- Scoop a bunch of pulp into the vat, mix, and swirl well;
- Dip the **mould** into the vat, scooping up the pulp, holding it level, **shaking** it until the water has drained through;
- Turn the mould, sans **deckle**, over onto a dampened felt on the **couching** stool.

Ta-da! A sheet of paper was made, waiting to be **pressed** and **dried**. It was, in fact, magical.

My first papers were soft, raggy, and thready, incompletely beaten with no **sizing.** However, they printed **letterpress** beautifully. I loved them. At the time, I was learning as many graphic processes as I could, including papermaking and bookmaking to expand my palette of choices as a student printmaker. Making my own paper allowed me to control the size, shape, weight, surface, and color I printed on. I was no longer restricted by available mould-made and machine-made paper. For me, there was excitement and liberation in this process.

Unfortunately, I quickly learned access to **paper mill** equipment was required. Making paper became an experience that had limits based on privilege and chance. At the time only a few institutions in the U.S. had these tools *and* someone knowledgeable enough to teach papermaking. Also, only a small number of private studios were producing handmade paper, either for sale or for creative projects. My privilege of attending a state university where papermaking happened to be an option blinded me to the reality that only a few select schools had such access. Time passed. I left U.W. where I had access to papermaking equipment. While I could still make prints, I could not make more paper without the necessary tools. Still, I knew the magic and could make paper when it was possible.

In 1980 I was hired by Arizona State University (A.S.U.) (https://art.asu.edu) to initiate a letterpress and book art studio within the printmaking area. Dr. Jules Heller was the Dean of the College of Fine Arts when I arrived. He wrote the first book on **contemporary papermaking** (Heller, 1978). His enthusiasm for the material and process helped acquire and equip basement rooms on campus with beaters, felts, and a **press**. Dr. Heller taught small groups of graduate students how to make paper and they eventually taught other students. However, when I started working at A.S.U., the paper mill was idle.

The paper mill remained vacant and unused during my first few years at A.S.U. During those years I established the letterpress studio, which later led to the book art publishing imprint of A.S.U., The Pyracantha Press (https://art.asu.edu/degree-programs/printmaking/pyracantha-press). Once my efforts found eager class enrollments and projects for the Press, I turned my attention toward the paper mill. I added papermaking to the curriculum with the keen approval of my administrators. Offering papermaking as a course forced me to quantify my knowledge, seek more sources of information, and prepare the content logically so students would understand papermaking better than I had when I first started my journey. I knew the magic would be there, but I wanted the students to understand the process and science of papermaking so they could be more creative and efficient. "Feel the sliminess" was no longer part of the curriculum. **Cellulose** fiber structure, **fibrillation**, and **hydrogen bonding** were added.

Over several years, my grasp of paper science and technique grew, aided by reading, attending conferences, meeting other artists who were making paper, and discussing materials and techniques. I also learned as the students learned. I adapted the traditional papermaking process to the Arizona desert and arid climate I was now living in. This included placing sheets that I pressed twice – once in felts from couching and once in **blotters** – into a forced-air **restraint dryer**, instead of the open-air drying techniques I used in Wisconsin. Sheets processed this way dried flatter with less **cockling**.

New fibers also became an interest for me. Although students and I made cotton rag paper to learn the basic steps, we used other plant fiber papers to further explore the process and biology. Nature provided us with many sources of cellulose besides cotton. The Sonoran Desert abounded with fibrous plants that could be used in papermaking, such as agave, yucca, Hesper aloe, desert spoon, mesquite pods, and even cactus skeletons.

Making Paper Mean Something

During this time, I did not consider papermaking to be meaningful to the art. Then one day in 1988 when my siblings and I were touring our uncle's Wisconsin farm for the last time before it was sold, I saw straw, jute feed bags, sisal bale twine, hemp ropes, and cotton seed sacks. At that moment, I realized I could make paper from all these fibers and create a keepsake of the family farm that was *of the farm* (Figure 1.1).

As a result of this experience, I saw how the ingredients of papermaking could be another element in the ideas and significance contained within the art. Pairing the printed image and word with the knowledge of the paper's substance gave the viewer a deepened aesthetic or intellectual experience of its story. It was not an application I would always use – some paper would be created solely as substrate, for a specific color, shape, or surface, as before – but the specificity and significance of the fiber content had become another possible element to explore.

Collaborations and Projects

Throughout my career as a teacher, printmaker, and papermaker, I often worked with other artists and writers. In 1984, A.S.U.'s printmaking area created the Visual Arts Research Studio (V.A.R.S.), in which we collaborated with invited artists to generate new print work. Faculty, as well as student assistants, examined and recorded the process of collaboration itself while we produced projects.

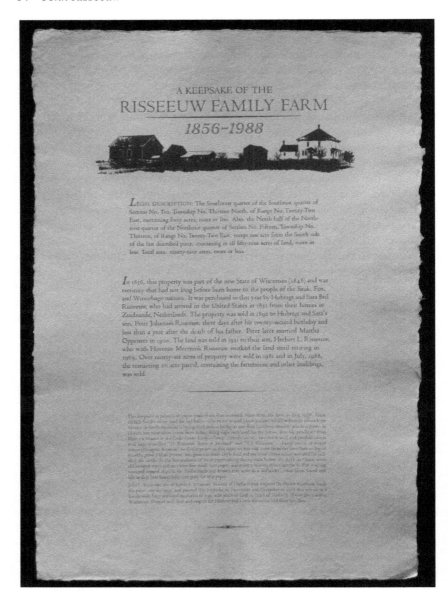

Figure 1.1 A keepsake of the Risseeuw family farm.

In addition, the Pyracantha Press took on numerous publication projects – books and **broadsides** – with writers and, later, scientists, biologists, and musicians. Collaboration or co-creation was second nature to many printmakers, and it certainly was part of my artistic practice.

The rest of this chapter features many of the collaborations and projects I have engaged in over the last 40 years. They frequently combined printed text, images, and content-specific fibers. The handmade paper also told powerful narratives to educate or bring awareness about current political and social issues.

Dance of Death, 1987

One of my early collaborations was a portfolio project that spanned several years. It was a contemporary take on the traditional *Danse Macabre* (*Dance of Death*). *Danse Macabre* has a long history stretching back into the Middle Ages when the ability to rationalize the value of a short, often miserable life with the fact of arbitrary and imminent death was difficult (Renauld, 2021). In each image, a person from any social class – the beggar to the Pope – was seen struggling with a skeleton, representing death, often with humor or irony. In the twentieth century, contemporary life and culture looked at death beyond the common disease and strife of the Middle Ages. Nuclear war, pollution, world hunger, oppression, the arms race, rainforest destruction, endangered species, and more were part of modern society's dance with death.

The collaboration invited artists, writers, songwriters, and essayists. Everyone contributed content with interviews, poems, songs, and artistic expressions to create a unique commentary about current life- and death-related topics. I responded by making paper with content-specific fibers, materials, and applications relevant to each contribution (Figure 1.2). Paper was then printed with the contributor's words or images to unite our work and messaging.

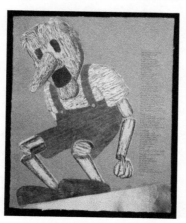

Figure 1.2 Grain.

Bill of Rights, 1991

In my role as director of The Pyracantha Press, my press assistant Daniel Mayer and I created Figure 1.3, a broadside commemorating the 1991 bicentennial of the U.S. Bill of Rights signing (Federal Register, 2021; National Archives, 2020). Challenges to individual rights seemed to be timely (Strossen, 1991) and the bicentennial was an opportunity to remind the public of the document's

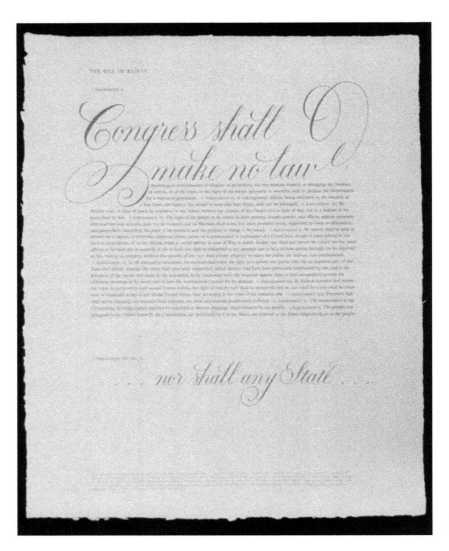

Figure 1.3 The Bill of Rights.

actual words. We collaborated with a law professor about the text and used his contention that these first five words were the most important: "Congress shall make no law." (National Archives, 2021, para. 6). Other nations' constitutions or charters often told the people what they could or could not do – the U.S. Bill of Rights began by telling the government what it *could not* do, an important distinction. These words were emphasized using late eighteenth-century style calligraphy printed on paper made from cotton American flags and blue jeans, which we believed were two quintessential American fiber sources. By using these resources, the paper's substance was connected conceptually to the content of the piece. We found that viewers having read the **colophon** and observed that the flags and jeans were made into paper demonstrated an immediate grasp of the broadside's physicality and significance.

Spirit Land, 1995

Purposeful fiber also became the starting point of another collaborative paper-making project for an exhibit and symposium at New York City's Cooper Union. This project was sponsored by the Dieu Donné Papermill (http://www.dieu-donne.org), a cultural institution committed to the collaborative and contemporary practice of papermaking. *The Art of the Matter: Dialogues between Master Papermakers and Artists* invited seven pairs of collaborators from around the country to participate. I was invited and then chose another papermaker/print-maker artist as my partner, making our collaboration the only one between two equal artists. Our back-and-forth concept development evolved into an **artists' book**, titled *Spirit Land,* which was created with content-specific paper from each of our states (University of Oregon, 1996).

My collaborator, Margaret (Peggy) Prentice, taught printmaking and paper-making at the University of Oregon. In addition, she co-founded the Twinrocker Paper Mill (http://www.twinrocker.com) in 1971, the first practical and success-ful hand paper mill in the U.S. since hand paper mills were closed in the early twentieth century (Baker, 2006). For this project, Peggy made paper from Or-egon plant fibers, such as cattails, seagrass, hemp, moss, fir tree needles, and cannabis. I made paper from Arizona plant fibers, such as Joshua tree, Spanish dagger, honey mesquite, green palo verde pods, and purple sage flowers.

Peggy printed color reduction woodcuts on our shaped papers, which re-vealed the different landscapes of each state (Figures 1.4 and 1.5). Inside the book, I printed lists of endangered plant species in both Arizona and Oregon (Arizona Native Plant Society, 2000; Oregon Natural Heritage Program, 2001). I also printed thoughtful and original poems about the environment written by Arizona writer Gary Nabhan and Oregon poet Kim Stafford. The book was held in a rough paper folder made from mixed fibers and dirt from both states. As readers handled the book's pages, they were given a tactile experience of the paper, bringing their attention to environmental concepts.

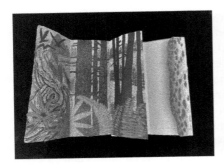

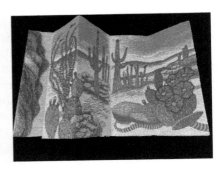

Figure 1.4 Spirit Land, Oregon side woodcut.

Figure 1.5 Spirit Land cover and Arizona woodcut.

Arms Trade/Victims, 1996

Arms Trade/Victims (Figure 1.6) made for *Hand Papermaking Magazine* (Vamp & Tramp Booksellers, 2017) turned out to be important in an unexpected way. The print contained facts about global arms sales such as a list of the top ten exporting nations and a list of weapons sold. The image was printed on paper made from recycled currencies of these countries mixed with clothing that represented victims of armed conflicts. Examples of the clothing included the following: 1) a cotton skirt worn by a South African woman murdered by an apartheid-era police force, which was sent to me by her sister; and 2) survivors, who were driven into southern Turkey after the Iraqi Army shelled their village, sent me clothing from Iraqi Kurds who were killed in the attacks.

In planning this piece, the process was an academic, intellectual exercise that translated into a visual product. This included researching and gathering lists of weapons traded or sold along with identifying dollar amounts by country. This inventory was then combined with images of money and death next to an accounting of victims. I designed the image as a **folio print** that must be opened to view. The colophon inside explained what created the paper. I found the power of touching the paper, once readers learned and knew about its content, had a strong emotive effect. The response for some people was immediate; they dropped the paper. The print communicated a tangible connection between weapons, money, and loss of life. For some viewers, the sum of this information became emotional and relational. There was power in this piece that I had not expected.

The Paper Landmine Print Project, 2001

Arms Trade/Victims became the basis for a new series as I became increasingly aware of worldwide landmine issues. I decided to make paper from the clothing of victims and survivors and then print images that would have both an

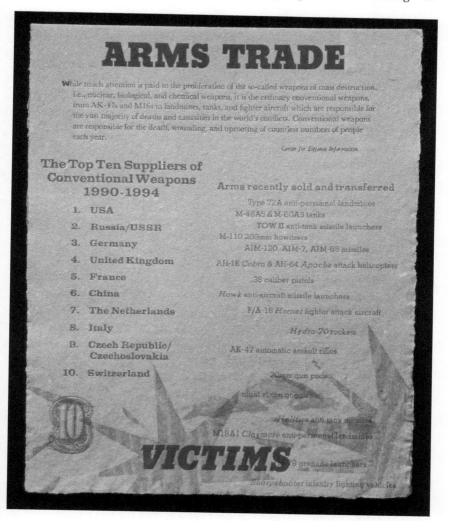

Figure 1.6 Arms Trade/Victims.

emotional and educational value. Again, the fiber to make the paper was not the actual clothing from landmine incidents. These donations were only representational to share the stories and educate others about the destructive realities of landmines.

When I began this project, the country of Cambodia, a nation the size of the state of Oklahoma in the U.S., had more than 60 landmine victims *a month*. When I traveled to Cambodia in 2002, the country was widely regarded then as the second most landmine-affected region in the world (Landmine Survivors Network, 2006; Mouly, 2001). Physicians for Human Rights (P.H.R.) recently noted:

> Between 1970 and 1990, the prevalence of landmines in Cambodia led to the highest percentage of physically disabled inhabitants in the world. The Cambodian conflict was the first war in history in which landmines claimed more victims – combatants and non-combatants – than any other weapon.
>
> (2022, para. 1)

In Phnom Penh, I spoke to a worker who removed landmines for the Mines Advisory Group (M.A.G.) (https://www.maginternational.org). The M.A.G. is a British non-governmental organization (N.G.O.) that located, dismantled, and re-moved landmines, cluster bombs, and unexploded devices in regions experiencing conflict (M.A.G., 2021). There I walked next to minefields to collect dried plants to use for papermaking. Then my next visit within the city was to Kien Khleang Rehabilitation Center. With support from the Vietnam Veterans of America (V.V.A.) (https://vva.org), they produced custom wheelchairs and prosthetics for landmine survivors. All the people employed in the organization were survivors themselves.

Upon returning home I felt overwhelmed with the amount of data I had collected and wanted to convey. To communicate the information from this trip, I designed one of my prints, *Map 'N Facts* (Figure 1.7) with a selection of facts within a map of the country. The printed image was influenced by the Oklahoma size comparison mentioned earlier, with a large "OK!" (the state's abbreviation) printed near the bottom. Hopefully, this element puzzled the viewers and drew their attention to the mix of landmine images and stunning details about Cambodia's landmine story.

The M.A.G. office in Cambodia connected me with a de-miner in northern Iraq where I learned they were clearing landmines left over from the 1980–1988 Iran-Iraq War (Dastbaz, 2020). With the information he forwarded, I did a print about the 3-inch Italian mine that was illegally exported to Iraq and used heavily in the north (McGrath, 1992). The print was titled *Ten Kilograms* (Figure 1.8) because that was the weight it took to trigger detonation: 22 pounds. This title seemed a straightforward way to connect viewers with the fact a child could set it off. The paper used for this print included shredded money of those nations using or manufacturing these mines.

My research also included a visit to Sarajevo, Bosnia. At the time of my visit the city was still recovering from the 1990–1995 war between former Yugoslav states. These regions were prolific producers of landmines before, during, and after their internal war (Williams, 1995). They used landmines from factories in Croatia, Bosnia, and Serbia and these devices frequently surfaced in other countries (United States Department of State, 1998). My visit included interviews at the Mine Action Center, Sarajevo University's Institute for Research of Crimes against Humanity (http://www.institut-genocid.unsa.ba), and interviews with

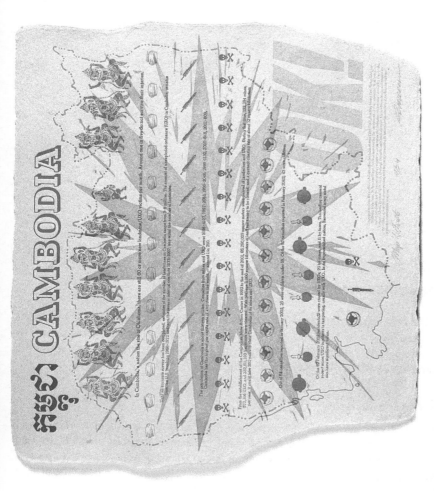

Figure 1.7 Map 'N Facts.

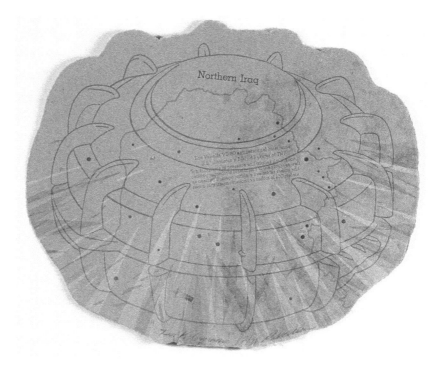

Figure 1.8 Ten Kilograms.

other individuals who provided a dizzying mixture of facts, insights, and ambi-
guities. Over 4,600 mine casualties in Bosnia and Herzegovina were honored in
Figure 1.9, *Ne Molim*. The dark paper and textures were intended to suggest the
darkness and lack of clarity found in the Balkan wars.

Survivor Stories

These travels not only helped me find more information about the history of
landmines, research their use, and bring more awareness to their devastating
effects, but I also met adult and youth survivors who were directly impacted.
Many shared their experiences and stories, as well as contributed to the project
by giving me significant fibers for making paper:

Cambodia

My knowledge of the people, problems, and history of landmines deepened when
I gathered personal stories at Phnom Penh's Cambodian Handicraft Association
(C.H.A.) for Landmine and Polio Disabled (http://www.cha-cambodia.org).

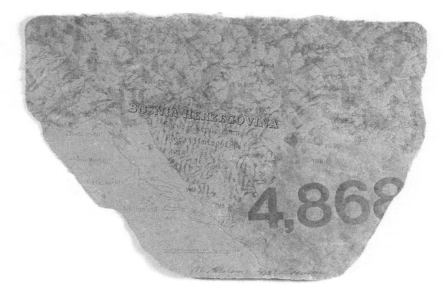

Figure 1.9 Ne Molim.

At the C.H.A., I spoke with women who were missing a lower leg from land-mine bombs. Some women gratefully donated articles of clothing for the project, perceiving my struggle to understand their trauma and the empathy I felt. Others were hesitant because they did not understand why this American was interested in their clothing and stories. *Strange Fruit* (Figure 1.10) was a print reacting to these experiences and the great contrast I felt in my visit: enjoying the people, scenery, and tropical fruits while learning about intimate landmine stories. I conveyed this in a collage of local fruits surrounded by a life-size Chinese landmine that had injured the women I met at C.H.A.

Mozambique

In Maputo, the capital of Mozambique, I interviewed landmine survivors and learned about the after-effects of 30 years of internal war in their country. My research uncovered a shocking list of nations in Asia, Africa, Europe, and North America whose landmines were found in Mozambique. In response, I printed *An African Story* (Figure 1.11). The print was **pulped** from donated clothing of survivors along with various African grass and plant fibers. I added money into the pulp from the countries that had landmines in Mozambique. I found the handmade paper becoming more variable and the fragmentation of the prints increasing, perhaps because of my growing dismay and knowledge about the widespread misery landmines caused.

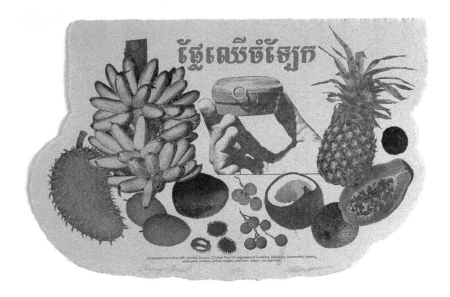

Figure 1.10 Strange Fruit.

Nicaragua

Through email contacts with organizations who remove landmines around the world, I received a red T-shirt from a landmine survivor in Nicaragua. With this piece of clothing, I created a print telling this man's story of being injured by a landmine on a coffee plantation where he worked. A second Nicaragua print (Figure 1.12) was created on paper that was made with the same man's shirt and burlap coffee sacks from the region. The paper also contained shredded

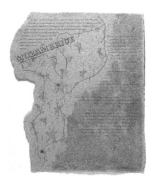

Figure 1.11 An African Story.

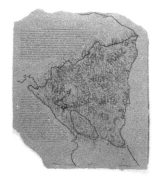

Figure 1.12 Minas no Mas.

money from Nicaragua, the U.S., and the Soviet Union, all participants in the 1981–1988 Contra War. This war left numerous landmines and explosive remnants in the area.

Angola

A United Nations Children's Fund's (U.N.I.C.E.F.) child protection services worker noted in 2001 about the Angolan Civil War (1975–2002):

> About 1 million Angolan children have lost one parent in the war and almost 300,000 have lost both parents. In addition, more than 1 million children across the country are believed to have no access at all to education and health facilities. In general, all children are direct or indirect victims of this war. Not a single family has not been affected.
>
> (IRIN News, para. 9)

My contacts at the V.V.F. provided me with a donated pile of landmine victims' clothing and currency from Angola. At the time, it was the third most heavily mined country in the world (Human Rights Watch, 1993; Landmine Survivors Network, 2006). Figure 1.13 was made from the pulp of these fibers, and it focused on the children of Angola who were significantly affected by the war.

Despite de-mining efforts, these problems still exist today. The children of Angola continue to be victimized by the ongoing use of landmines. The unique colors, shapes, and sizes of landmine devices have often enticed children to pick up and play with them (Afrol News, 2022).

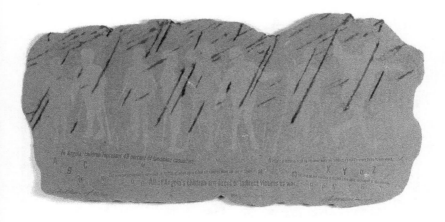

Figure 1.13 Children of War.

BOOM! Artist Book, 2011

Gathering context and content for the Paper Landmine Print Project and those affected by landmine use was an amazing expansion of my knowledge and awareness, as well as an appalling illustration of human cruelty. After 12 years of research, trips, and the production of 15 prints, I realized the project could continue for years since there were 62 countries with landmine problems. To bring my own efforts to a close, an important next step for me was to create an artist book, *BOOM! A Summary of the Paper Landmine Print Project* (Risseeuw, 2011). This book provided an overview of the work and updated the information I had collected. Placed on irregular-shaped pages, images identified the affected countries with chaotic compositions that conveyed the violent disorder of life after war. The 12-foot-long accordion structure extended and compounded the knowledge of the lives lost and spent in Angola, Bosnia, Cambodia, Iraq (Figure 1.14), Nicaragua, (Figure 1.15), and other countries. As a

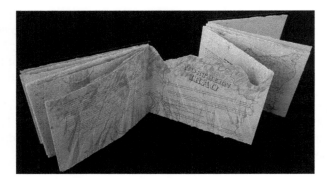

Figure 1.14 BOOM!, Iraq spread.

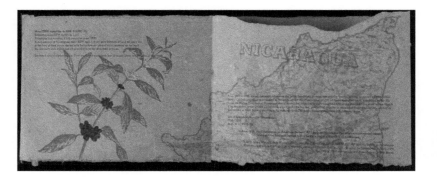

Figure 1.15 BOOM!, Nicaragua spread.

two-sided accordion book, the backside pages were filled with additional facts and quoted sources, as well as woodcut and textural imagery.

The edition of 30 prints were primarily purchased by university library collections and the Library of Congress, sometimes with prints from the project. By editioning the work, I hoped it would be widely disseminated, making it available for many years to come. Institutions often highlighted new acquisitions or promoted such holdings for public use, newsletters, articles, and exhibits. The placement in public collections was important to bring attention and access to landmine issues through the book and prints. Searches for the content by the public and scholars curious about the subject would direct them to view the work at nearby locations.

The art was eventually exhibited in 91 venues within the U.S., Netherlands, Bulgaria, Canada, Italy, Japan, Scotland, and South Africa. The exhibition included ten solo shows. The project was featured in 25 publications (Cochran & Potter, 2014; Rose & Eliot, 2019; Rossman, 2007) and I gave 34 lectures and presentations. In the same way that public collections provided access to this work, the exhibits, writings, and talks served to inform a wider public about the astounding global issues of landmines. Each viewer, many of whom were college and university students, gained new knowledge and awareness about conflict and the human issues that remain because of the detritus of war.

The prints were in editions of between 20 to 40 copies, depending on how much pulp I was able to beat for a particular print. Each print sold for $500. The remaining copies of the book sell for $2,000. The proceeds from these sales were and continue to be donated to humanitarian organizations that help landmine survivors, remove landmines, and have supported this project. Over $30,000 has been donated. Consequently, researching the scourge of landmines and generating financial support and public awareness through print sales for victim assistance and N.G.O. action was a natural consequence of my own engagement with the world.

Progress has been made. Charitable organizations have helped thousands of victims and cleared thousands of acres of previously mined land. However, I am always hopeful for more as landmine problems remain. The Landmine Monitor from the Nobel Prize-winning International Campaign to Ban Landmines (I.C.B.L.) (http://www.icbl.org) reported in 2021 that threats to civilians from landmines and other explosive remnants of war (E.R.W.) continued to be high and of great concern. Although the numbers of casualties in some formerly high-risk nations have reduced, the number of landmines planted in other nations has risen.

Conclusion

Papermaking and advocacy have sparked and expanded ideas toward social engagement that I rejected or only briefly employed at the beginning of my career. My undirected path drifted into this rewarding world of **socially engaged art** (**S.E.A.**). Collaborative art production led me into creation by interconnection;

the joys of minds meeting minds to solve tasks and problems with human discourse. Greater works of art and thought were achieved by multiple interactions than individual effort could manage. It was through collaboration and teaching that I learned the most throughout my career in prints, paper, and books. I found greater arenas of thought and deeper applications of work for a larger community.

Content-specific papermaking has become embedded in my creative library. It surfaces, when necessary, with a metaphorical hand that reaches out and slaps the viewer upside the head to say, "Pay attention here!" I am humbled to have contributed something to the field that has extended well beyond my career to better lives and opened people's eyes to the magic in paper.

References

Afrol News. (2022). Demining Angola annually costs U.S. $88 million. http://www.afrol.com/articles/15335.

Arizona Native Plant Society. (2000). Rare plant guide. U.S. Government Publishing Office. https://aznps.com/rare-plants.

Baker, C. (2006). *Hand papermaking in the twentieth century*. [Conference presentation]. Guild of Book Workers Standards of Excellence Seminar, New York, N.Y. https://guildofbookworkers.org/content/journal-centennial-issue-cathleen-baker.

Cochran, J., & Potter, M. (2014). John Risseeuw: Prints on paper. In J. Cochran & M. Potter (Eds.), *Social paper: Hand papermaking in the context of socially engaged art*. Columbia College.

Dastbaz, J. (2020, February). Explosive remnants of Iran-Iraq War still claiming lives and limbs. RUDAW Media Network. https://www.rudaw.net/english/middleeast/iran/09022020.

Federal Register. (2021). Commission on the bicentennial of the United States Constitution. https://www.federalregister.gov/agencies/commission-on-the-bicentennial-of-the-united-states-constitution.

Heller, J. (1978). *Papermaking*. Watson-Guptill.

Human Rights Watch. (1993, February). Landmines in Angola: An African watch report. https://www.hrw.org/reports/pdfs/a/angola/angola.932/ango932full.pdf.

IRIN News. (2001). IRIN focus on children of war. https://www.thenewhumanitarian.org/report/22192/angola-irin-focus-children-war.

Landmine Monitor. (2021, November). International Campaign to Ban Landmines – Cluster munition coalition. http://www.the-monitor.org/media/3318354/Landmine-Monitor-2021-Web.pdf.

Landmine Survivors Network. (2006). Landmine facts. http://landminesurvivors.org/what_landmines.html.

McGrath, R. (1992). Hidden death: Land mines and civilian casualties in Iraqi Kurdistan. Human Rights Watch. https://www.hrw.org/reports/1992/iraq.

Mines Advisory Group International. (2021). What we do. https://www.maginternational.org/what-we-do.

Mouly, I. (2001). A national mine action institution: The Cambodian mine action center. *Journal of Mine Action, (5)*1, 8–12.

National Archives. (2020, August). The Center for Legislative Archives. Bill of Rights. https://www.archives.gov/legislative/features/bor.

National Archives. (2021). America's Founding Documents. The Bill of Rights: A Transcription. https://www.archives.gov/founding-docs/bill-of-rights-transcript.

Oregon Natural Heritage Program. (2001). *Rare, threatened, and endangered plants and animals of Oregon.* Institute for National Resources Publications.

Physicians for Human Rights. (2022). Where we work | Cambodia. https://phr.org/countries/cambodia.

Renauld, M. (2021). *Danse Macabre*: The allegorical representation of Death. The Collector. https://www.thecollector.com/danse-macabre-middle-ages-danse-of-death.

Risseeuw, J. (2011). *BOOM!: A summary of the paper landmine print project.* Cabbagehead Press.

Rose, J., & Eliot, S. (2019). *Companion to the history of the book.* John Wiley & Sons.

Rossman, J. J. (2007). *The activated page: Handmade paper and the artist's book.* The Jenny-Press.

Strossen, N. (1991). Americans' Love-hate relationship with the Bill of Rights celebrating the bicentennial of the Bill of Rights in honor of the centennial of the Detroit College of Law: Essay. https://digitalcommons.nyls.edu/cgi/viewcontent.cgi?article=1159&context=fac_articles_chapters.

United States Department of State. (1998). Hidden killers 1998: The global landmine crisis. [Archive]. https://1997-2001.state.gov/global/arms/rpt_9809_demine_ch3i.html.

University of Oregon. (1996). Artist books at the University of Oregon Libraries. *Spirit land/Nabhan, Stafford, Prentice, Risseeuw.* Cabbagehead Press.

Vamp & Tramp Booksellers. (2017, December). Catalog.

Williams, J. (1995). Landmines: A global socioeconomic crisis. *Social Justice, 22*(4), 97–113.

Zinn, H. (2007). Artists in times of war. *CLCWeb: Comparative Literature and Culture, 9*(1), 1–9. http://www.doi.org/10.7771/1481-4374.1033.

2 Pulp, Pull, Press, and Print

Engaging with Papermaking in Community Art Workshops

Raoul Deal

This chapter describes the papermaking experiences of community art students conducting intergenerational papermaking workshops in a variety of contexts. In partnership with youth groups, senior centers, and community organizations, student artists help create opportunities through papermaking for participants to manage the process of aging, empower violence prevention in youth, and support grieving mothers of gun violence. The chapter outlines strategies for utilizing the medium as a means of personal and collective transformation, creating a space of shared vulnerability, cooperation, and collaborative art-making.

About Community Arts

As art has moved from traditional museums and galleries into alternative community settings, theorists and practitioners have grappled with new terminology to describe and analyze the different ways in which art now operates. Community-engaged art, a collaborative and interdisciplinary practice, has been measured largely by the degree to which it was useful and meaningful to the communities it served. It often blurred the lines between professional practices such as ethnography, public health, social work, and various types of pedagogy.

Community-engaged art also has roots in the social and political movements that formed in Europe and the Americas over the past 150 years (Finklepearl, 2013; Goldbard, 2005; Helguera, 2011). For example, after the Watts Rebellion of 1965, artists from Watts Towers Arts Center in Los Angeles provided creative activities to community residents processing their trauma after the violent neighborhood destruction (Carter, 2003). Noah Purifoy, founding director of the Center, and Watts artists redefined their roles as creators and moved toward a concept of community involvement, activation, and engagement. They created opportunities for artists to participate in programs geared toward improving the lives of people who lived in the area. Purifoy noted that, for centuries, art-making had been considered a mysterious and inaccessible process, an activity often intended for the elite. His criticism of the exclusivity of art was robust. In his words, "I wanted to tell the world that this is untrue; that we are blinded by

DOI: 10.4324/9781003216261-4

this concept and that therefore no one would try to analyze the creative process in terms of its applicability to something else" (Smith, 2012, p. 169). By introducing the art-making process to Watts' neighborhood residents, they hoped to democratize it.

To democratize art required establishing a new criterion and a different way of valuing it. In speaking about the Watts Art Movement, and the shift toward community engagement, Carter (2003) noted "The artist in these settings is expected to be a caring person committed to developing a community of thought and collaboration where the art produced functions as a cohesive, healing force" (p. 8). Centering accessibility to the creative process as a core guiding principle differentiated community-engaged art from other art forms, which simply appeared in communities. Community-engaged artists were often facilitators who sought to uplift and share power through participation in collaborative, creative experiences. What was gained through the *process* of these expressions mattered more than the completion of any polished or finished product. As highlighted in this chapter, papermaking allowed a similar collaborative, creative process.

About Community Arts and Papermaking at U.W.M.

The Community Arts Program at the University Wisconsin Milwaukee (U.W.M.) (https://uwm.edu/arts/art-and-design/community-arts) has been structured as a Bachelor of Arts program to provide students with ways to explore and use art at the service of others, and towards the "common good" (Velasquez et al., 1992). Students in the program have experimented with strategies to address cultural, political, social, and environmental concerns. They used art processes that were often collaborative, multidisciplinary, and accountable to the communities with which they worked.

I was first exposed to papermaking in 2014 when I answered a call from Max Yela, the Director of Special Collections at U.W.M. Golda Meier Library. He invited me and community art students to participate in a hands-on workshop with the Peace Paper Project. The Project was in Milwaukee that week teaching how to **pulp** fibers, make paper, and create prints. All of this was new to me, but I was attracted by the prospect of working with and learning from this international community arts organization. The Project also shared the U.W.M. Community Arts Program's basic goals and values.

I invited several artists and cultural workers from around Milwaukee to share in that first experience. Participants learned the mechanics of pulping and **pulling** sheets of paper and how to create shapes and images through **double-dipping**, stenciling, and **pulp printing**. In addition, it was inspiring to learn about the Peace Paper Project's strategy of collaborating with art therapists to use papermaking as therapy. Working with a variety of groups, such as veterans, refugees, and survivors of sexual violence, participants transformed significant fibers into paper to process memories and emotions through symbolic expression (Peace

Paper Project, 2022). Peace Paper Project Founder, Drew Matott, described the experience of cutting up the **rag** as a moment of sharing space and stories, and participants bonded as they carried out project activities. Pieces were pulped in a **Hollander beater** and turned into paper, which individuals used for drawing, painting, and journaling.

Finally, students were fascinated with how resourceful Matott had been in finding ways to accommodate the specific needs of the communities where he facilitated papermaking. For instance, in communities without electricity, he had created an option for powering the Hollander beater with a bicycle. He simply replaced the bike's back tire with a plastic belt so the beater could be operated by anyone who could pedal. For the students in the workshop, it was a remarkably efficient and popular activity (Figure 2.1).

For many of us, the workshop was transformative. U.W.M. was inspired to purchase an **Oracle Hollander beater** to offer papermaking experiences to students on a regular basis. Since then, we have offered a papermaking course through the college's Peck School of the Arts (P.S.O.A.). Additionally, our papermaking facilities are often used by instructors and students for class projects

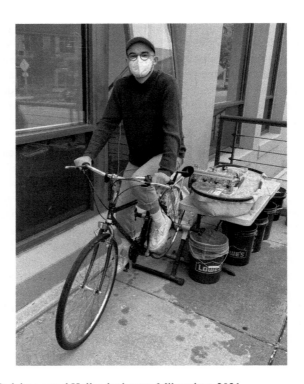

Figure 2.1 Pedal-powered Hollander beater, Milwaukee, 2021.

and self-directed individual experimentation. This has resulted in the development of new skills, interests, and approaches to art-making that many students continued to build on as they moved beyond the walls of the institution.

Collaboration and Social Engagement

Collaborative art practices are carried out with different levels of social engagement. Helguera (2011) proposed the following tentative taxonomy of **socially engaged arts (S.E.A.)** and its connection to participation: a) nominal, b) directed, c) creative, and d) collaborative. In the Community Arts Program, the work was carried out using *collaborative participation*, where everyone shared responsibility for both structure and content. As part of university coursework, these projects were limited by time and experience, with their success often depending on power-sharing and co-creation strategies. For example, it was particularly exciting when participants engaged in creative dialogue and critical examination that led to mutual ownership. Everyone felt capable to reproduce the activity with others.

Papermaking as Collaboration

Papermaking was well suited to this level of collaboration. Both students and community participants often felt empowered by the process. Students brought **moulds** and **vats** to Hyde Park Art Center (https://www.hydeparkart.org) to work with young artists and Jim Duigan, Associate Professor in Art Education at Depaul University. Duigan is the Founder of the Stockyard Institute (http://www.stockyardinstitute.org), a community-based project that has engaged high school students throughout Chicago in the arts (DePaul University, 2022). Duigan described how the Stockyard Institute first provided central Chicago youth living in the Back of the Yards neighborhood with opportunities to explore the daily challenges they faced. The conversation with youth was intense and centered around four topics: work, land/sustainability, resilience, and gender/sexuality. U.W.M. students explored these themes in collaborative ink drawings that were later transferred to the paper they made on the roof of the Hyde Park Art Center. Once back in Milwaukee, the paper was **pressed** and **dried** and their drawings were completed. The paper that was produced embodied not just the collaborative process of creating it (Figure 2.2), but also what was learned on the trip about art as a tool for overcoming personal hardship and addressing society's ills.

Watching students work through the entire project made me think more about what might be possible in future projects. The thrill of making paper and the meaning behind the process was clear. Using papermaking to explore common experiences through collaborative writing and drawing created another layer of meaning.

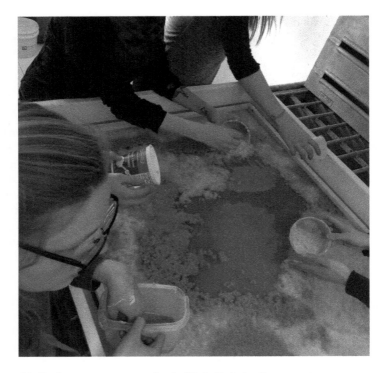

Figure 2.2 Students prepare paper for the Hyde Park Art Center project.

Papermaking as Community Building

Papermaking was uniquely capable for building community because it was collaborative and gratifying. In addition, the process was simple enough to yield results regardless of previous exposure to the medium. Papermaking was integrated into all U.W.M. community art classes to build friendship and camaraderie in each cohort. Once students learned the basics, they were anxious to explore more, either as a service-learning activity with community partners or in collaborative projects with the entire class. Whether working in schools, neighborhoods, or simply with classmates, projects were conceived with the key purpose of strengthening bonds with peers and building community with the groups with which they worked. Here are examples of these experiences:

Student Artists in Residence

One way students used community-engaged papermaking was through participation in Student Artist-in-Residence (S.A.I.R.) (https://uwm.edu/community/students/student-artist-in-residence), a program developed by theater artist,

U.W.M. educator, and eldercare specialist, Anne Basting. Basting has been crafting opportunities for elders to experience art and creativity as they age. S.A.I.R.s, some of whom were matched to live and work in senior communities for an entire year, were placed around the city. Within these communities, student artists carried out art activities with the residents.

Jessica was an S.A.I.R. assigned to Eastcastle Place, an assisted living facility on Milwaukee's near north side. When Jessica began her work at the site, she observed challenges within the resident community. One was a general lack of agency. Many people were afraid of making art and did not believe they were equipped. Additionally, there were different ability levels and some residents experienced low vision and limited hearing. Since it was important to carry out inclusive activities that anyone could participate in, Jessica discovered she had to adjust the process. Although making paper was tactile, visually stimulating, and it looked "fun" to do, the process was wet, noisy, messy, and smelled. This made it less attractive than expected for some residents. The following recollection from Jessica illustrated some of the engagement difficulties she had in the beginning:

> The morning of [the workshop], one woman left a note outside my door that just said she couldn't make it, and also that I needed to make my invites bigger for readability next time. I stuck that one in my paper bag to be pulped. A few people told me in passing why they couldn't come. I noticed one woman (who had cried at my first meeting because she didn't know what I was talking about) was pacing outside the room as we made paper, and later she stopped in, to scope things out. Still, she wasn't interested in trying. She said, "I just want to be able to do something that I'm able to do".
>
> (personal communication, December 16, 2021)

Once the activities began, however, most residents became excited and engaged (Figure 2.3). It became a rich, satisfying process that had an element of surprise and instant gratification. Jessica commented further:

> You know it's almost like a ripple effect – someone might try it first and maybe someone who's not as brave to try it kind of just sees what's going on, and you get sucked in, and I feel like that's the same thing that happened when I did papermaking with Eastcastle Place.
>
> (personal communication, November 6, 2021)

Ultimately, two of the residents became so engaged, they invested in their own moulds and **deckles** and began making paper with their neighbors. They held papermaking sessions to make cards and they experimented independently

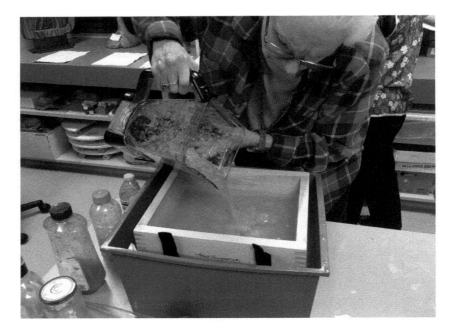

Figure 2.3 Marilyn adds pulp to the vat.

with the medium. Residents sold these cards at the holiday market, inspiring fundraising as well. In her final reflection about the event, Jessica wrote:

> There's like an alchemy that happens where you just see the shift in the people that are a part of it. Even though it took a lot of effort, it was worth it to see people get so into the process. I remember feeling that way when I first did it, so that's all I could ask for. It was awesome seeing Judith (pseudonym) using a cane with one hand and holding a blender of pulp in the other.
> (personal communication, December 16, 2021)

Project Ujima

In the fall of 2018, students were part of an ongoing collaboration between U.W.M.'s Community Arts Program and Project Ujima, a violence prevention program at the Children's Hospital of Wisconsin (https://childrenswi.org). The program provided services to families who had experienced trauma from violence. P.S.O.A. supported the work through the school's Kenilworth Community-Engaged Arts Initiative and provided space, expertise, and expanded university resources to carry out the work (McManaman, 2018; University Wisconsin Milwaukee, 2019).

In anticipation of a week-long Project Ujima workshop, students prepared the materials. They made large moulds and deckles out of wooden silkscreen frames, cut new **couching** cloths, and coated stretched silkscreens for burning text and images Ujima youth artists would create later. Students also had the opportunity to experiment with pulping and making paper themselves. For most, it was the first time they had experienced papermaking.

The workshop was ambitious and challenging. To finish in the time allotted, we secured the participation of two community-engaged artists from the city. Images were co-crafted with the support of Paul Kjelland, a local interdisciplinary artist and project organizer with Justseeds (http://www.justseeds.org), an artist cooperative committed to social, environmental, and political engagement. Paul helped the youth create photographic self-portraits and separate them into layers for two-color printing. Text for the portraits was explored under the guidance of Milwaukee hip-hop culture artist and TRUE Skool (http://www.trueskool.org) Co-Executive Director, Fidel Verdin. He helped the youth develop or find self-affirming phrases to transfer onto their paper. We hoped experimenting with lyrical phrases would tap into pre-existing interests the youth might have in their spoken word and hip-hop culture. Given that the Peace Paper Project was also in the area, on an annual U.S. tour to colleges and universities, Drew Matott came to assist us on-site.

During the workshop, two processes were used: a) pulp printing (Figure 2.4), a technique we had learned from Matott, and b) conventional silk-screening. Silk-screening was selected to achieve a crisper resolution for the text we were printing, but its use also exposed the group to its potential for creative entrepreneurship. Silk-screening has been commonly used both as a medium for self-expression, and to generate income through the sale of T-shirts, posters, and other popular items. Due to the nature of the workshop, we hoped the youth might create slogans or images that could be used in this way. The benefits of social entrepreneurship for young people have also been found to be neurological. Research has noted how adolescent brain development aligns well with youth social entrepreneurship (Kruse, 2019). The medium was motivating, and exciting, and the youth were alive and engaged.

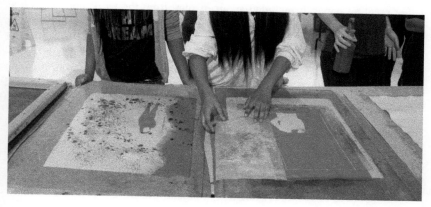

Figure 2.4 Pulp printing on the project's second day.

Ujima staff members were supportive of the proposed activities. The staff members' main goal was that the youth had the opportunity to experiment with creative self-expression. The impact of making art was sorely needed for many of the youth, as local opportunities for creative self-expression were limited. They clearly enjoyed making paper and creating the images and messages they printed on the sheets. Having time to connect and make art that day was beneficial and meaningful.

One of the surprising outcomes of the project was the stress relief and joy the workshops brought to Project Ujima's crime victim advocates, who attended the initial planning sessions and were present at the face-to-face meetings with the youth. Instead of having this group solely as support for the youth, we invited them to engage in the project. Several advocates expressed how much they appreciated the chance to experiment and learn using these creative activities.

Everyone was encouraged to bring in pieces of clothing that had special meaning or were significant to them. However, only Jackie, one of the Ujima crime victim advocates, chose to do so. Her own family had been fostered in the program after experiencing trauma from violence. Jackie brought a bag of neckties and an African hat that had belonged to her deceased father. Jackie shared that her father wore this hat every year during Black History Month. Her father also had been a local Minister/Elder of the gospel and had acted as a mentor to countless Black boys. Among other things, he taught them how to tie a necktie. Jackie spoke of how her father believed this was an important skill, useful to all who hoped to rise and succeed in their lives. He did this, she said, as an act of caring and compassion. These personal items carried the weight of her father's legacy as a beloved community member and teacher. Jackie described how turning his hat and ties into paper was calming, brought her peace, and honored her father in a way that gave her a sense of healing from the grief of his passing (personal communication, November 8, 2018).

The culminating event was a celebration of the time participants spent together creating paper. It included an art display from the workshop, as well as papermaking activities for participants' friends and families. For the gathering's preparation, I asked one of Ujima's crime victim advocates to work together with a community arts student to create an exhibit statement describing the experience. The pair summarized the workshop in lyrical, rhythmic phrases that reflected the complexity and excitement of the week, and hinted at the profound ideas that had emerged:

Would you offer up your favorite piece of clothing to serve a greater purpose?
Articles of clothing, gathered by the traveling Peace Paper Project, once
*   belonged to individuals that made it out of _____,*
that we all have felt once before.
Nothing becomes beautiful without pressure; remember, it produces diamonds.
Let that marinate!

Days ago, this gallery was movin' and groovin' as if we were building the
Fiserv Forum. Four days, eight hours, nine kids and seven staff from
Project Ujima,
Eight Community Arts students, two UWM staff, and four working artists.
With everyone buzzing around with purpose, we trusted the process of
diving into it together, as messy as it was bound to get.
We "jazzed up" the pulp mixtures with our hands, dipped our moulds in, splash!
Jump back. Water on the flo.
Pulp saturated screens drip until it is ready to press and blot.
Here is when we made the choice, accepting the challenge to tell you the truth.
How we feel about judgment, why we feel the need to run to a better education,
Why we feel our futures can't blossom.
If I want to continue making art, who will support me?
"We've got moms, dads, kids, and wives, too."
Project Ujima, Peace Paper Project, and U.W.M. Community Arts
Welcomes and appreciates your support.
"Judgment becomes permanent justice."
"I feel best helping people."

Mothers Against Gun Violence

Students from the Community Arts Program often collaborated with other P.S.O.A. departments. I was approached by Portia Cobb, Associate Professor in Film, Video, Animation & New Genres, to collaborate with Mothers Against Gun Violence (M.A.G.V.). M.A.G.V. is a support and advocacy group in Milwaukee for survivors of gun violence. Founder Debra Gillispie had facilitated interviews of survivors and their families to be used for a theater production based on their stories. In addition, she was interested in using therapeutic art with her group and educating the public about gun violence. I described the papermaking workshops the Community Arts Program did with Project Ujima, and we began planning an event for M.A.G.V. Debra proposed the workshop could be an opportunity for participants to bring clothing significant to their deceased family members and turn it into paper.

Debra was purposeful in inviting participants likely to be open and trusting of one another. All the women had joined the workshop to support one another, and each considered the opportunity to be another step along their own healing. Some of the women also helped others on their journeys with life after loss. One of these participants was Colette. Colette worked as a coach with We Loved and Lost (http://www.welovedandlost.com), a company she started after losing her son to gun violence. Another participant was Gloria. Gloria created Robert's Way, a GriefShare group, to honor her son (Lauren, 2019). Additionally, Carrie was a community leader and advocate. She worked to combat domestic violence and the disappearances of young Indigenous women. Carrie provided support services for families of victims and survivors.

During the first day of the workshop, the main objectives were as follows: a) to build trust and community among the group, b) teach the basics of papermaking, and c) invite participants to experience the therapeutic properties of the medium as they proceeded through each stage of the day's activities. Everyone had the opportunity to state why they had come, and their expectations for the workshop. Survivors shared whatever they were comfortable with, and everybody listened attentively and with compassion. The stories were emotional and raw. They were hard to share and hard to hear. There was laughter and there were tears. As the afternoon progressed, the women began the process of cutting up the article of clothing they had brought (Figure 2.5).

At the end of the day, the mothers contributed messages they wanted to turn into pulp printing screens for the next session. Some were tied to their group's advocacy objectives, such as "We take a stand against gun violence" or "We take a stand against domestic violence." Others alluded to ways of coping with their loss: "Walk it out" and "You can do anything you want to do." A couple of the families chose highly personal phrases that only held special meaning for them. For instance, "Queen Diva" was how one mother's son always referred to her. "Scott Girls 4 Life" was another such phrase. The whole family adopted it as a declaration of unity and strength. Finally, there were words such as family, forgiveness, honor, purpose, and the positive affirmation, "You too will grow from here!"

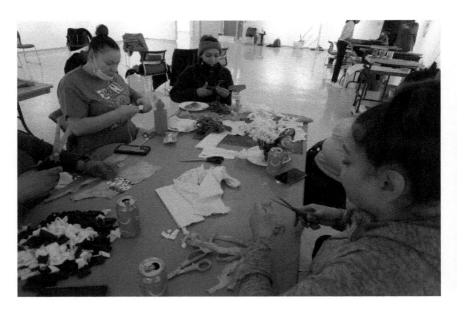

Figure 2.5 M.A.G.V. workshop participants prepare their deceased loved ones' clothing for pulping.

On the second day, after everybody had pulled sheets of paper, and experimented with **pulp painting** and printing, the significance of the process was unfolding and becoming increasingly powerful. Colette stated:

> The pieces of material being cut were the pieces that I had to put my life back together after losing my son. With every snip, I had to be willing to cut up what I didn't ask for [my loss]. Then those pieces were pulped together through a process. I got a bag. This was symbolic of my loss. And in that bag, it was very mushy. And again, it was like the process of healing after my loss … and going through the actual water to make sure that all of the material was dissolved enough to make paper […] I felt connected to my son and like we're going to make something together. When I touch this, I feel as if, um, not so much that [my son is] here, but that this workshop was a place where I could just feel as if we're one.
>
> (personal communication, April 9, 2022)

During the project, student facilitators balanced the gravity of the themes addressed, with the need to help participants experiment with the papermaking processes. This was especially true when interacting with the youth, who were playful, but fully aware of the workshop's intent. For example, one 10-year-old participant was especially active in the process. He loved everything about it, and he was quick to get his hands in the pulpy water. He made more paper than anyone and he could describe the activities in detail. He later recounted the experience of separating the fibers and putting the **sizing** in the vat where the mould would be dipped. He explained its purpose:

> So then when we make […] the paper, it won't like rip easily. Don't fall apart when you touch it or something. […] More like, a boa constrictor grabbing prey, […] like it gets tighter and tighter, so it won't get out easily. So then when it dries, you can paint and draw [on it].
>
> (personal communication, April 9, 2022)

He also understood the project's deeper meaning. When asked what he would tell others about the workshop, he said, "Don't worry. It's okay – that you missed your family or even lost it, it's okay. [This] will be a symbol that you can always have of them even in the afterlife."

One of the mothers spoke about what it was like to do the workshop with her young daughter. She recalled her daughter saw her cry as she shared a memory of her brother. Her daughter sensed what her mother felt and cried as well.

> I don't know, I guess for a second… I felt like I was in her place because like when we lost my brother and my mom was hurting, I felt like I was feeling my mom's hurt, but I wasn't trying to overshadow what she was feeling during that process. And I felt like [my daughter] was kind of doing the same for me.
>
> (personal communication, April 9, 2022)

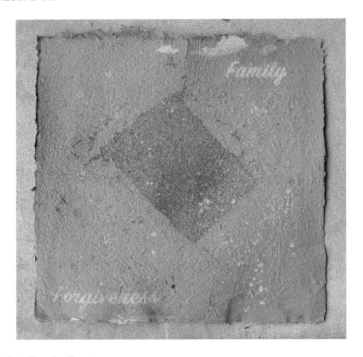

Figure 2.6 Family, Forgiveness.

As the second day continued, some of the paper that was made required nothing further. For example, Alicia simply centered a small blue rectangular sheet diagonally in a larger, lighter background, gently splattered with color. She placed the words family and forgiveness along the edges (Figure 2.6).

It was heartening to witness how the papermaking process nurtured each participant. Nobody wanted it to end. Two of the mothers suggested the papermaking workshop be made available in numerous Milwaukee communities where it could reach others grieving the loss of a loved one. Another mother asked if it would be possible to create an image of her son and print it on the paper she had made. We added another workshop to accommodate her request.

During this third workshop as the women entered the room, silkscreens were lined up along the windowsill with images of their loved ones ready to be printed on their paper. It was a powerful moment. Colette explained, "It's like you took something that had been lost to us, and you brought it back to life!" (personal communication, May 19, 2022). Additionally, Gloria added text to accompany the portrait she made of Robert (Figure 2.7). Before printing it, she said just two things. "Leave the holes in the paper – I'm feeling the funk …" and "don't change how I spelled *sonshine* – I want it just like that" (personal communication, April 19, 2022).

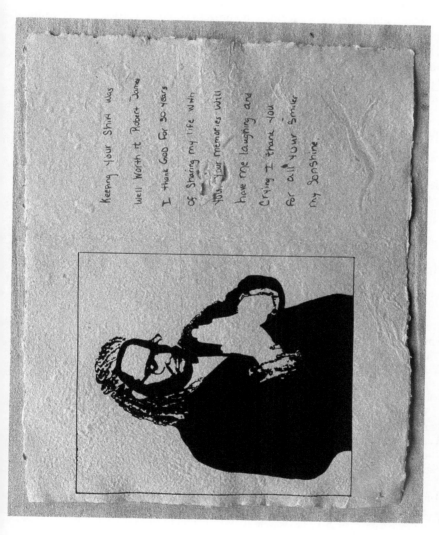

Figure 2.7 Completed image of Gloria's son Robert James.

Conclusion

Since the first workshop with the Peace Paper Project in 2014, papermaking has become an integral part of community arts education at the Peck School of the Arts. Although the simplicity of the medium was attractive, the experience was profound. Furthermore, we learned the process could be carried out with little or no previous experience, and by people of different ages and abilities. We also realized that providing access to papermaking activities in community arts workshops enhanced the lives of elders and youth, aided in processing grief and trauma, and brought students and workshop participants together with a common purpose to experience the transformative power of creative self-expression.

References

Carter, C. L. (2003). Watts: Art and social change in Los Angeles, 1965–2002. Haggerty Museum of Art.

Depaul University. (2022). Taking art to the streets. https://www.depaul.edu/distinctions/Pages/to-the-streets.aspx.

Finkelpearl, T. (2013). *What we made: Conversations on art and social cooperation.* Duke University Press.

Goldbard, A. (2005). *Art/Vision/Voice: Cultural conversations in community: A book of cases from community arts partnerships.* Columbia College.

Helguera, P. (2011). *Education for socially engaged art: A materials and techniques handbook.* Jorge Pinto Books.

Kruse, T. P. (2019). *Making change: Youth social entrepreneurship as an approach to positive youth and community development.* Social Justice and Youth Community Practice Series. Oxford University Press.

Lauren, A. (2019, April). "This doesn't go away": When your child is murdered, grief is only the beginning. Cycles of violence: A Journal Sentinel special report. Milwaukee Journal Sentinel. https://projects.jsonline.com/news/2019/4/11/when-your-child-is-murdered-grief-is-only-the-beginning.html.

McManaman, A. (2018, April). Peck School initiative brings new artists, energy to INOVA Gallery. U.M.W. report. https://uwm.edu/news/peck-school-initiative-brings-new-artists-energy-to-inova-gallery.

Peace Paper Project. (2022). Papermaking as art therapy. http://www.peacepaperproject.org/arttherapy.html.

Smith, R. C. (2012). *The modern moves West: California artists and democratic culture in the Twentieth Century.* University of Pennsylvania Press.

University Wisconsin Milwaukee. (2019, March). U.W.-Milwaukee Community Engaged Scholars Network (C.E.S.N.) Newsletter. https://uwm.edu/community/wp-content/uploads/sites/239/2019/03/March-2019-Community-Engaged-Scholars-Network-Newsletter_Draft-2.pdf.

Velasquez, M., Andre, C., Shanks, T., & Meyer, M.J. (1992). The common good. *Issues in Ethics, 5*(2), 45–60.

3 Paper as Praxis

Steven Kostell and Meadow Jones

Introduction

Thank you for turning your careful attention to this page. You hold in your hand a physical object, a book bound of paper, made, and manufactured for the printing and **pressing** of this text. Based on the ideas of the art of papermaking, this chapter addresses the process of papermaking as a form of social engagement. The content presents the praxis, poiesis, and practice of making handmade paper, and explores the types of variations that can occur.

In 2014, The Columbia College Center for Book and Paper Arts in Chicago, Illinois, offered an exhibition on papermaking titled *Social paper: Hand papermaking in the context of socially engaged art* (Cochran & Potter, 2014). As part of the exhibit, key moments were charted about papermaking as an arts or craft practice and the cultural phenomenon of **socially engaged art (S.E.A.).** The timeline covered about 120 years, beginning with the development of Roycroft Studios and Mountain House in 1895 to the exhibit's present day. This thorough investigation provided a careful, neatly defined series of relationships, providing the viewer with accessible knowledge about S.E.A. development in hand papermaking. The delineation of these intersecting elements showed the tidy outcomes of complex coordination. This chapter contributes to this intellectual and cultural lineage by revealing the messy machinations of interconnections, collaborations, and untidy transformations that are part of hand papermaking as a social practice.

The history of papermaking can be viewed as a history of humanity. Paper, humble and proud, has served as the vehicle for content communication: a memory made manifest, a container of knowledge, and a technology of telling. Paper became currency in our hands. It is the book where this chapter was written and printed. Paper has been the surface of the walls around you, and the grid on your car's head gasket. Paper can be seen as being ubiquitous and often invisible – mass-produced from the forests of trees and rivers.

Papermaking shaped the process of industrialization, from villages working together using traditional methods to huge, modern facilities producing and

DOI: 10.4324/9781003216261-5

shipping the paper around the world for everyone to use. To make paper by hand is both to return to the old and to create new, to make form from the formless.

Hand papermaking has experienced a renaissance concomitant with the current do-it-yourself (D.I.Y.) movement. D.I.Y. as third-wave craft also references the third-wave feminist movement (Budge, 2016, 2019). This moment in papermaking may relate to the re-emergence of handmade craft production in the U.S. The medium can also be viewed as a continuation of the feminist D.I.Y. craft movement, sometimes referred to as **craftivism** (Greer, 2014). Occasionally referred to as a "feminine" medium (Cochran & Potter, 2014), papermaking is a practice of craft instead of artistic production. Craft as community-building is within the tradition of feminist pedagogy, as an artist-initiated, non-hierarchical, and decentered social action. It is both traditionally and contemporarily a practice that is resource-rich and dependent, requiring and using much capital, including human capital. In publicly engaged pedagogical arts, the papermaker takes this practice out of the studio, the audience out of the gallery, and participatory arts activities out into open spaces.

What is Praxis and Social Practice?

Political theorist Hannah Arendt (1970) articulated the distinction between poiesis and praxis, and between action and work. Poiesis and praxis "is the function … of all action … to interrupt what otherwise would have proceeded automatically and therefore predictably" (pp. 30–31). Action and work, in contrast, are defined as making the predictable occur. These concepts can be used to frame the complex components of artist-initiated social practice in hand papermaking. According to Arendt, acts of speech, to speak, and to be spoken to are necessary components of constructing the polity. Joining in communal conversations has activated political action and articulated the personal, making the public, private. Thus, a change in the polity leads to political change. Accumulation of personal narratives in an open venue can lead to social change. In the case of inserting narratives in the paper, artists have actively extended the practice of hand papermaking into the community. Engaging the public through material transformation facilitates an interrelationship between human and non-human interactions (Kester, 1999). The process of making the arts object embedded within social narrative becomes a type of public political participation (Jones, 2019). S.E.A. as a contemporary art practice encourages action toward social and political change (Murry, 2012).

Systems of Interaction: People, Place, and Materials

Imparting the tradition of a handicraft process has continued through formal training in higher education, serving as a critical link in the preservation of the craft as an art form. The nature of disseminating education has been a hierarchical form of interaction. While the studio apprenticeship model exists, access to opportunities was afforded to those who knew about them. Additionally, there were few pathways to acquire this knowledge through workshops and learning intensives.

Each method provides unique entries into the craft with an emphasis on creative approaches or production. The way training is passed through papermakers is through experiencing the process and thereby understanding the myriad variables one can encounter. As new practitioners emerge and seek to expand practice into open spaces, the process has changed and continues to change as it moves from the institution and into the public.

People

The hand papermaking process allows for persons to connect with materials, a negotiation between human and non-human. Locating the practice of papermaking in a public space puts the process of making on display as a spectacle, converting everyday materials into a fibrous liquid **pulp**, to then be transformed back into a solid. The process is wet, physical, time-consuming, and collaborative by tradition. This form of social participation promotes the emergence of community, an opportunity to come together around a common experience (Bishop, 2006). Likewise, artists collaborate with the community to bring voice to social issues, preparing in advance of the project and bringing necessary materials and tools from the studio to the site. This coordination of materials and place invites community members to participate in a system of interactions where they contribute to the material process and the resulting objects. Through this material-based production, individuals choose how and when to become involved in the process, impacting artistic outcomes through co-production.

Kiff Slemmons – Arte Papel

In a *Hand Papermaking Magazine* interview (Kostell, 2015) with Kiff Slemmons, the artist described the symbiotic relationships between people, place, and material interconnected through handmade paper. At the time, Slemmons recounted her 12-year collaboration with the papermakers of Arte Papel in Oaxaca, Mexico. She described working with the skilled papermakers to develop papers that would be converted with the Arte Vista Hermosa jewelry makers (Figure 3.1). Slemmons noted the economic opportunities developed because of this collaboration. By sourcing the local fiber stream and engaging the skills and labor of the artists, they were interacting in a mutually beneficial system. Finally, the emergent qualities contributed to the local creative economy and community.

Jillian Bruschera – The Mobile Mill

The Mobile Mill (https://themobilemill.tumblr.com) is an activist-focused project that engages directly with communities through a pop-up model. Artist Jillian Bruschera created "a transportable space able to interact between edges"

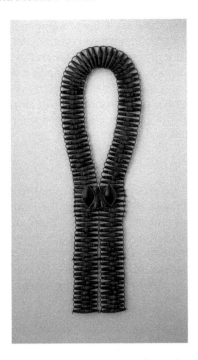

Figure 3.1 Red and Black Cover, 2019. Inked paper, silver, ebony, painted chicken bones, leather (pin is detachable), 24" × 7" × 1/2". Photo by Kiff Slemmons.

(Martin, 2015, para. 12) as "a way to actively engage in a variety of communities and dialogues" (para. 8). Due to its modular and transient design, the project offers the opportunity to participate in the papermaking process to any interested person in any available location (Figure 3.2). In addition, the Mobile Mill engages communities as a process of ongoing documentation by converting recycled material to paper. This approach to hand papermaking production provides the necessary resources to the public. The public then generates paper that visually and aesthetically records the event and reflects the diversity of persons who participated.

Places

When making paper by hand in public participatory environments, people were introduced to the craft process through a reflexive tradition (Oliver & Badham, 2013). A community of practice developed through engaging with materials and one another (Sanders-Bustle, 2020). This form of intentional learning was guided by a self-interested motivation and a curiosity about the affected ways of non-human power relationships (Bennett, 2010). By relocating the art

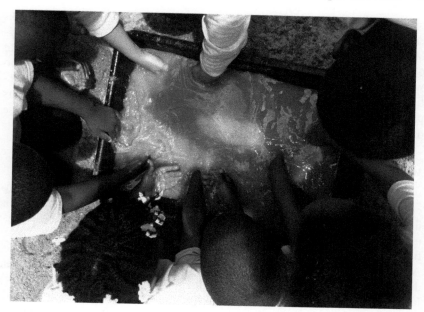

Figure 3.2 Prior to forming sheets, children from the community gather around a charged vat. Photo by Jillian Bruschera.

of hand papermaking into the larger public, communities were exposed to socially engaged methods and material production. This helped gain insight into the complex relationships between socioeconomic structures. Participants also contributed to social and cultural capital within the community and learned to envision new realities (Bourdieu, 1986). The specificity of each hand papermaking event led to a new aesthetic object and a unique experience. The interaction of varying fibers made for distinct kinds of paper, colors, textures, and tones. Equally, variations in stakeholders and narratives changed the experience of the participatory process, lending to a sense of thing-power (Bennett, 2010), as the innate ability for material to enter dialogue with the individual actors.

Historically, papermaking production spanned interior and exterior spaces, activating both non-built and built environments as sites for production. These spaces were most aligned with paper production growing to an industrial scale. As traditions of handicraft production declined, some lab-scale equipment found its way into academic programs, community art centers, artist co-ops, and creative entrepreneurial ventures. Academic programs gave rise to a slow and steady generation of artist practitioners. Professional organizations, including the North American Hand Papermakers (N.A.H.P.) (https://www.northamericanhand-papermakers.org) – formerly known as the Friends of Dard Hunter – and the International Association of Hand Papermakers and Paper Artists (I.A.P.M.A.)

(https://www.iapma.info), bridged the distant communities of hand papermakers. They also promoted sharing of experiences, techniques, and formalized relationships in an emergent community of practice (Wenger, 1998a). This form of situated learning focused on *doing* with a group of individual persons, who were not always local to one another, but who were interested in common activities. Members sought to master the application of papermaking, explore its processes, and share with others their insights and knowledge gained from those discoveries (Lave & Wenger, 1991; Wenger, 1998b).

Materials

With the continued growth of practitioners, a demand steadily grew for economically feasible resources, which in turn spurred entrepreneurial innovation. This innovation included the redesign and production of hand papermaking equipment at a smaller and more affordable scale. These changes increased locations for hand papermaking, decentering it from the institution into the public. Additionally, conversations altered the craft from private establishments to open discourse. Sites for socially engaged papermaking (Cochran & Potter, 2014) included the following: a) within the academy (academic/educational programs), b) institutions (museums/galleries/special collections), c) social non-profits (planned/targeted spaces) and community art spaces (site-specific), d) public spaces (pop-up sites/public intervention), and e) telematic broadcasts (mediated/interactive). As a formal academic or educational program, artists **activated** the medium of hand papermaking as social interaction with materials and compelling situational practice. Both applied intentional community interaction via coordinated partnerships (Lawton, 2019) and by engaging with communities through public intervention (de Vere & Charny, 2017).

This approach linked communities to places, both urban and rural, as city lots or agricultural plots. These sites for engagement emerged as community-facing, inviting the local public into the participation of material relation, connecting fibers to place, and routing a standard narrative through a shared experience. As artists increased access to this practice away from the academy, it became vital to develop strategies that supported and liberated papermaking from the institution and to develop cultural capital by expanding access to resources beyond the studio. However, for "access" to occur, it was not enough to ensure the availability of a resource; people also needed to be able to utilize what was available (Ribot & Peluso, 2003). To accomplish this goal required decentralizing the assets to provide resources to those who did not have access to them for use-making and the opportunity to experience an "intra-action" (Barad, 2007, p. 33) with materials in community with others. Toward this end, when working within communities an acknowledgment of the complexity of relationships (Wenger, 1998a) becomes critical for developing connections and trust through collaboration (Rutten et al., 2018).

Through the D.I.Y. maker's ethos, an artist-led approach to social practice establishes the project, guides the process, and leads participants through the process by imparting technical and practical knowledge. Such "inter-action" encouraged story sharing in relationship to materials and others, created community through empathy, and formed trust through collaboration (Emery & Bregendahl, 2014; Lawton, 2019). This kind of engagement was built on the sharing of personal knowledge as a journey through materials, practical experience, and resulting growth in human capital (Becker, 1993; Budge, 2019).

Similarly, additional models of collaboration may occur between the paper artist and the public, and these interactions can be initiated by the artist or a co-facilitator. The dominant model in higher education or studio apprenticeship is traditionally hierarchical, teacher to student. With the practice removed from the institution, interactions between the public and facilitators were decentralized, although the resources of the institution could be used. Public participation in the papermaking process added new variables to the practice, altering both the artistic process and the resulting artifact that symbolized the event. As the physical and emotional participation between the maker and material occurred, it allowed for an anthropomorphic reflection through realizing a material vitality (Bennett, 2010).

Narrative, Experience, Transformation

Risk and failure are inherent in hand papermaking processes. Although an iterative process, the duration of the project allows for multiple attempts toward controlling the variables. Proficiency is created with each attempt to form a sheet of paper. This process yields an increasingly familiar experience. For most participants, having no experience with the craft is humbling. This allows for both introspection while working toward technical knowledge and retrospection. The process also allows time to reflect on being with materials and cultivating a holistic empathy, as a kind of practical knowledge (Schwartz, 2000). The method of making paper provides opportunities for potential failure. Sometimes this happens when out of rhythm with the process, or by not understanding or knowing the behaviors inherent to materials (Sormani et al., 2019; Wu, 2021). Through community interaction and collaboration, iteration is continuously modeled, encouraging perseverance in continued participation.

The process of making paper is akin to the process of becoming a papermaker. It requires iterations, repetitions, familiarity, and endurance. The endurance is physical (lifting and heaving heavy, wet, sodden **moulds** soaked with pulp) and psychological (repeating the same practices endlessly towards a perfection that is ever elusive). As the **hydrogen bonds** form the sheet, social bonds are created that build community. In the case of papermaking, the binding process is essential for making a solid sheet that can endure external and internal forces, as well as endure tensile and shear forces for tolerating other physical manipulations, such as the imprint of a text.

This metaphor readily carries over into the attachments made in the social dynamics of hand papermaking. In fostering community, bonding happens through the sharing of individual experiences; it is established collaboratively and shared collectively through the papermaking process. Relational narratives are embedded into the material through physical and emotional making. Introducing the public to hand papermaking can become the focus of attention, knowledge, exploration, and group sharing, characteristic of a community of practice. This, in turn, weaves fibers of connectedness through otherwise loosely woven meshes of present-day social life.

Fresh Press

In 2011, one of the chapter authors, Steven Kostell, along with Eric Benson, created Fresh Press (https://www.freshpress.studio), an agrifiber and agri-waste papermaking lab. Fresh Press was created to facilitate collaboration between farmers, artists, designers, and academics under the auspices of a land-grant institution of higher education (Figure 3.3). The initial aim was to drive a conversation about ways regional **fibersheds** could help revitalize a slowly dying Midwest manufacturing industry. The project focused on community-centered

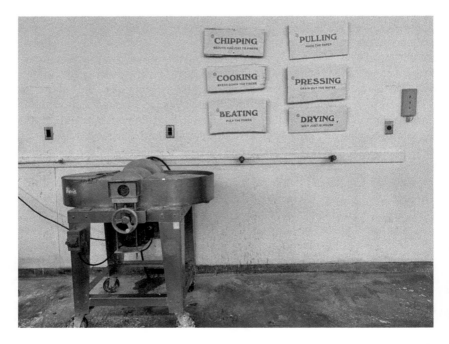

Figure 3.3 The Hollander beater awaits workshop participants. Signage describes the stages of paper production in the Fresh Press studio. Photo by Eric Benson.

engagement by connecting people to place. This brought an awareness of agricultural production along with an understanding of biomass as a value-added resource. A model was established by converting plant fiber through hand papermaking.

Capitalizing on the agricultural landscape and the assets of the prairie, with its abundantly available fiber sources, the team hoped to reduce agricultural waste and to redirect extractive practices toward regenerative processes. To accomplish this, Fresh Press established an active and ongoing **paper mill** used for a wide range of projects. Emphasis was placed on social practice through community engagement, often focusing on topics of environmental degradation versus regeneration. The project also capitalized on the local fibershed resources to achieve entrepreneurial independence in material production. Of particular importance was taking the process back to the farm as an on-site demonstration of papermaking. This included highlighting the circular nature of the material production, such as growing, harvesting, processing, and the transforming of material. One's relationship to the landscape was embedded in the narrative and constructed through the experience of place-based making.

Panty Pulping

In 2011, Margaret Sheppard (Mahan), Drew Matott, and Gretchen Miller established the Peace Paper Project, which explored ways to engage communities in dialogue with contemporary social issues. One aspect of the project sought to engage communities in conversation about consent culture by inviting the public to bring their undergarments and participate in **Panty Pulping** (Figure 3.4). Considered a personal garment, underwear as a source material carried a certain shock value, which stirred interest and speculation as to how people would initiate participation. Through making paper, participants converted underwear to heighten social discourse around topics about sexual violence, sexual autonomy, and mutual respect (Jones, 2016).

In the process of **pulping** these clothing fibers, the participants actively and freely contributed personal material into the communal batches of pulp. Garments were combined and pulped for fiber to be shared with others in the community. A modified bicycle-powered Hollander beater was used. Participants took turns exerting physical labor to pulp the fibers for others to yield as paper. For some participants, the bodily interaction was viewed as radical and liberating. The activity conjured an elevated level of excitement over the duration of the event. For others, it became an opportunity to integrate their trauma, share stories and inform the critical discourse around consent culture, toward social innovation.

These two distinct projects demonstrate the diversity of fibers, as intentions and outcomes, while using similar material processes and artistic actions. Fresh Press relates to issues of the environment, restorative practices, labor, and capital. Panty Pulping relates to an opportunity for intervention into social

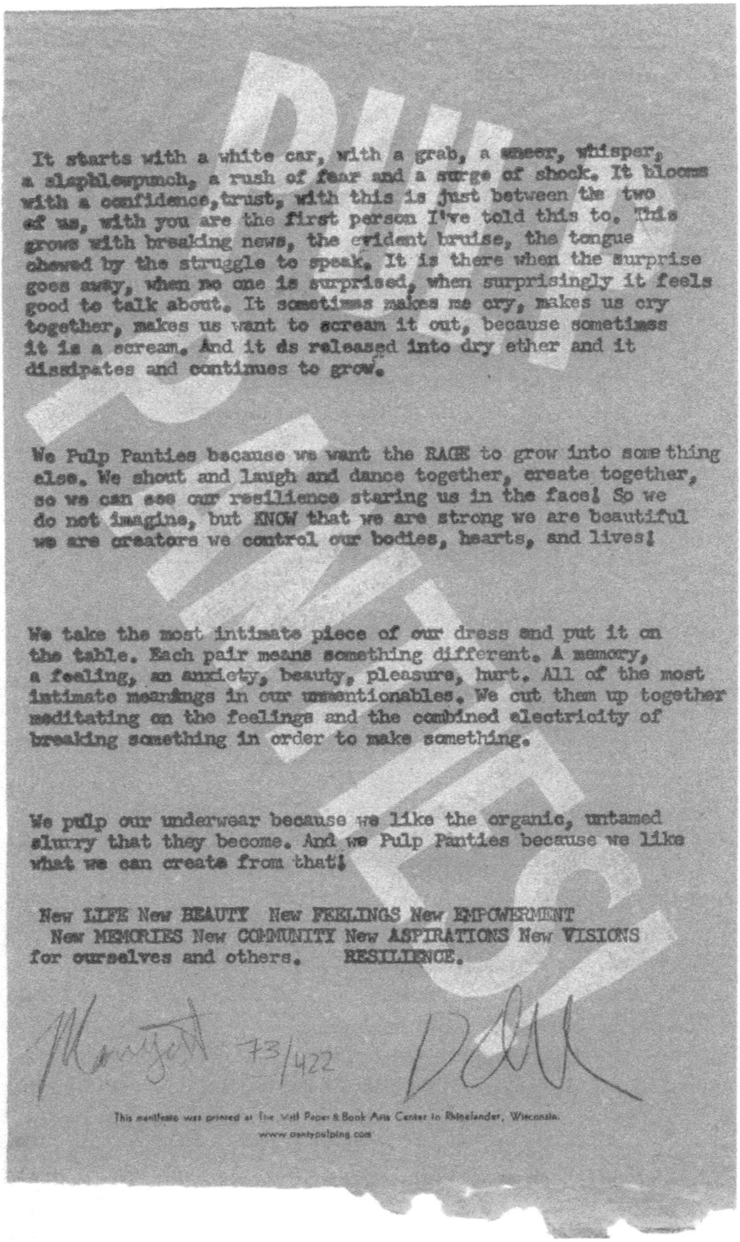

It starts with a white car, with a grab, a sneer, whisper,
a slap blow punch, a rush of fear and a surge of shock. It blooms
with a confidence, trust, with this is just between the two
of us, with you are the first person I've told this to. This
grows with breaking news, the evident bruise, the tongue
chewed by the struggle to speak. It is there when the surprise
goes away, when no one is surprised, when surprisingly it feels
good to talk about. It sometimes makes me cry, makes us cry
together, makes us want to scream it out, because sometimes
it is a scream. And it is released into dry ether and it
dissipates and continues to grow.

We Pulp Panties because we want the RAGE to grow into something
else. We shout and laugh and dance together, create together,
so we can see our resilience staring us in the face! So we
do not imagine, but KNOW that we are strong we are beautiful
we are creators we control our bodies, hearts, and lives!

We take the most intimate piece of our dress and put it on
the table. Each pair means something different. A memory,
a feeling, an anxiety, beauty, pleasure, hurt. All of the most
intimate meanings in our unmentionables. We cut them up together
meditating on the feelings and the combined electricity of
breaking something in order to make something.

We pulp our underwear because we like the organic, untamed
slurry that they become. And we Pulp Panties because we like
what we can create from that!

New LIFE New BEAUTY   New FEELINGS New EMPOWERMENT
  New MEMORIES New COMMUNITY New ASPIRATIONS New VISIONS
for ourselves and others.   RESILIENCE.

This manifesto was printed at The Wolf Paper & Book Arts Center in Rhinelander, Wisconsin.
www.pantypulping.com

Figure 3.4 Panty Pulping Manifesto. Photo courtesy of the Richard F. Brush Art Gallery, St. Lawrence University, Canton, New York.

violence toward a more just society. Both afford the opportunity for engagement with materials, for a better understanding of symbiotic relationships to place and each other, and for building communities of practice. Meanwhile, artists coordinate and facilitate a space for nurturing an intimacy of the relationship between objects and individuals (Barad, 2007). This association with materials acknowledges an emotional connection – woven into the myriad layers of cultural connections – through the act of making. For each project, to make is to innovate – to move from one state to another – and to affect and experience transformation through co-production.

Conclusion

Through work, the world and all its constituent components, people, places, and things are transformed (Arendt, 1970). This is the praxis of social practice and papermaking. Making paper can be seen as distinct from other craft forms in that we are making the vessel for narratives embedded within the object. With the making of paper, we are manifesting form from formlessness. It is a process of negotiations between a person's hands and the **slurry** of fibers. This transformation takes a material framed as intrinsically valueless and gives it value through the process of making and it makes visible its value through co-making. With papermaking in public spaces, a co-production of both the objects produced and the process experienced can occur. Socially engaged practices of hand papermaking build community by connecting or facilitating relationships between people, place, and material. Transformation of fibers is enabled through co-production that results in a shared social narrative.

Acknowledgments

The authors would like to thank the friend-scholars who read drafts-in-progress of this work, including Dr. Sharon Irish, Dr. Hong-An Wu, Boyd Porter-Reynolds, Edward Dietkus, Michael Gaiuranos, and Dr. Michael Brün. Their insights contributed to the improvement of this chapter.

References

Arendt, H. (1970). *On violence*. Houghton Mifflin Harcourt.

Barad, K. (2007). *Meeting the universe halfway: Quantum physics and the entanglement of matter and meaning*. Duke University Press.

Becker, G. S. (1993). *Human capital: A theoretical and empirical analysis, with special reference to education*. University of Chicago Press.

Bennett, J. (2010). *Vibrant matter: A political ecology of things*. Duke University Press.

Bishop, C. (2006). *Participation: Documents of contemporary art*. M.I.T. Press.

Bourdieu, P. (1986). The forms of capital. In J. G. Richardson (Ed.), *Handbook of theory and research for the sociology of education* (pp. 241–258). Greenwood Press.

Budge, K. (2016). Teaching art and design: Communicating creative practice through embodied and tacit knowledge. *Arts and Humanities in Higher Education, 15*(3–4), 432–445. https://doi.org/10.1177/1474022215592247.

Budge, K. (2019). The ecosystem of a makerspace: Human, material and place-based interrelationships. *Journal of Design, Business & Society, 5*(1), 77–94. https://doi.org/10.1386/dbs.5.1.77_1.

Cochran, J., & Potter, M. (2014). *Social paper: Hand papermaking in the context of socially engaged art.* Columbia College Chicago Center for the Book and Paper Arts.

de Vere, I., & Charny, D. (2017, August). Social innovation in the curriculum: A model for community engagement and design intervention. In *Proceedings of the 21st International Conference on Engineering Design*, Vol. 9: Design Education, Vancouver, Canada.

Emery, M. E., & Bregendahl, C. (2014). Relationship building: The art, craft, and context for mobilizing the social capital necessary for systems change. *Community Development, 45*(3), 279–292. https://doi.org/10.1080/15575330.2014.903986.

Greer, B. (Ed.). (2014). *Craftivism: The art of craft and activism.* Arsenal Pulp Press.

Jones, M. (2019). Archiving the trauma diaspora: Affective artifacts in the higher education arts classroom. *Marilyn Zurmuehlen Working Papers in Art Education 2019* (1), 1–14. https://doi.org/10.17077/2326-7070.1516.

Jones, R. E. (2016, October). Peace Paper Project turns underwear to art at local colleges. Seven Days. https://www.sevendaysvt.com/LiveCulture/archives/2016/10/16/peace-paper-project-turns-underwear-to-art-at-local-colleges.

Kester, G. (1999). Dialogical aesthetics: A critical framework for littoral art. *Variant, 9*(1), 1–21.

Kostell, S. (2015). Esteem the giver: Q&A with Kiff Slemmons. *Hand Papermaking Magazine, 31*(1), 16–19.

Lave, J., & Wenger, E. (1991). *Situated learning: Legitimate peripheral participation.* Cambridge University Press.

Lawton, P. H. (2019). At the crossroads of intersecting ideologies: Community-based art education, community engagement, and social practice art. *Studies in Art Education, 60*(3), 203–218. https://doi.org/10.1080/00393541.2019.1639486.

Martin, L. (2015, December). *8 questions for a traveling paper maker.* https://makezine.com/2015/12/09/interview-jillian-bruschera-papermaking-mobile-mill.

Murry, M. (2012). Art, social action, and social change. In C. Walker, K. Johnson, & L. Cunningham (Eds.), *Community psychology and the economics of mental health: Global perspectives.* Palgrave. http://dx.doi.org/10.13140/2.1.1291.1049.

Oliver, J., & Badham, M. (2013). Re-presenting the everyday: Situational practice and ethnographic conceptualism. *Laboratorium, 5*(2), 149–165.

Ribot, J., & Peluso, N. L. (2003). A theory of access. *Rural Sociology, 68*(2), 153–181. https://doi.org/10.1111/j.1549-0831.2003.tb00133.x.

Rutten, K., Van Beveren, L., & Roets, G. (2018). The new forest: The relationship between social work and socially engaged art practice revisited. *The British Journal of Social Work, 48*(6), 1700–1717. https://doi.org/10.1093/bjsw/bcx118.

Sanders-Bustle, L. (2020). Social practice as arts-based methodology: Exploring participation, multiplicity, and collective action as elements of inquiry. *Art/Research International: A Transdisciplinary Journal, 5*(1), 47–70. https://doi.org/10.18432/ari29488.

Schwartz, D. T. (2000). Empathy, interpretation, and judgment: The case for art. In D. T. Schwartz (Ed.), *Art, education, and the democratic commitment* (pp. 67–110). Springer. https://doi.org/10.1007/978-94-015-9444-8_4.

Sormani, P., Bovet, A., & Strebel, I. (2019). Introduction: When things break down. In I. Strebel, A. Bovet, & P. Sormani (Eds.), *Repair work ethnographies: Revisiting breakdown, relocating materiality* (pp. 1–30). Palgrave Macmillan.

Wenger, E. (1998a). Communities of practice: Learning as a social system. *Systems Thinker, 9*(5), 1–10.

Wenger, E. (1998b). *Communities of practice: Learning, meaning, and identity.* Cambridge University Press.

Wu, H. A. (2021). Where's the time to care? *The Temporal Politics of Caring for Educational Technologies. Research in Arts and Education, 4*: 164–189.

Part II

Papermaking as Art Therapy

4 Adaptations and Modifications for Therapeutic Hand Papermaking

Genevieve S. Camp, Amy Bucciarelli, and Amy Koski Richard

This chapter presents unique adaptations to hand papermaking methods for three distinct projects: a) a group process within an eating disorder treatment center; b) the development of a modular approach for bedside work with people hospitalized for medical conditions; and c) the integration of hand papermaking activities into a school curriculum for students with developmental delays. Symbolic and therapeutic aspects of hand papermaking are also discussed.

For the co-authors, the connection between hand papermaking and art therapy began much like editors Matott and Miller described earlier – a series of "unexpected encounters," leading to "defining moments." After seeing the Peace Paper Project (n.d.) in action at a papermaking conference, artist Amy Richard sought partners to host their visit to Gainesville, Florida. A colleague serendipitously connected Richard with medical art therapist Amy Bucciarelli. Familiar with the watery, potentially messy process, Bucciarelli joked, "If you can figure out how to bring hand papermaking into a hospital, I'm on board!"

Soon after, these individuals found themselves hosting a week-long series of community Peace Paper Project events. These included a day-long workshop at the hospital where Bucciarelli worked. Hospital staff, caregivers, and patients (who were mobile, and had doctor approval), made paper in an outside hospital garden. Iconic symbols of Western medicine and illness, hospital sheets, gowns, and masks were **pulped** and transformed into artful pages of hope.

Genevieve Camp, an art therapist at the hospital-affiliated eating disorder center, attended the event. Intuitively, she saw that cutting, tearing, and pulping clothing patients had outgrown, as they healed and restored weight, could be therapeutically transformative. Camp's experiences that day inspired her to ask Bucciarelli and Richard to help introduce hand papermaking to patients who were being treated for severe eating disorders. This request marked the beginning of numerous collaborative workshops with varied populations. One example included teaching hand papermaking to other therapists in partnership with

DOI: 10.4324/9781003216261-7

the prestigious Dieu Donné Papermaking Studio (http://www.dieudonne.org) for the Expressive Therapies Summit, an annual creative arts therapies conference in the U.S. (https://summit.expressivemedia.org).

The ongoing partnership provided fertile ground for innovating, mentoring one another, and contemplating the therapeutic benefits of papermaking. For example, Camp experimented with a multi-step papermaking project for patients with eating disorders, Bucciarelli developed modular kits for bedside papermaking in a hospital, and, lastly, Richard adapted what she had learned from graduate studies in paper and book arts to serve public school students with learning disabilities. The following essays describe the strategies, adaptations, and insights that developed through these unexpected encounters with hand papermaking.

Hand Papermaking in an Inpatient Eating Disorder Program

Genevieve S. Camp

Eating disorders (E.D.s) are complex psychological–medical conditions that result from a combination of genetic, behavioral, and psychosocial factors (Seubert & Virdi, 2019). In general, E.D.s are characterized by dysfunctional eating behaviors (e.g., restricting, binging, purging) and the tendency for body weight or shape to unduly influence self-worth (American Psychiatric Association, 2013). These disorders can be challenging to treat because the E.D. behaviors function to regulate the nervous system (Scatoloni, 2019). E.D. behaviors can be understood as an adaptive way (through a small or large body) of providing comfort, soothing, numbing, distraction, predictability, structure, protection, or safety, and even a sense of identity. Additionally, they can be a cry for help; a form of self-punishment, self-cleansing, or self-purification; a way of avoiding intimacy; and a way to blame oneself instead of blaming others (Costin, 2007).

Working with E.D.s involves exploring unique and personal stories of how and why the disorder developed while also helping situate body image concerns within the larger societal context. In *The body Is Not an Apology*, Sonya Renee Taylor (2018) described the concept of *radical self-love* as necessary to counter the "constant barrage of shame, discrimination, and body-based oppression" communicated through popular media (p. 7). Acknowledging that Western beauty standards (i.e., fair-skinned, youthful, thin, toned, able-bodied) are rooted in race, class, and gender prejudice (Strings, 2019) can lead patients to recognize that healing their relationship with their body is a radical act of self-love, and part of collective healing. Hand papermaking can contribute to recovery, by offering participants an experience of the body as a resource for personal and collective healing, rather than an obstacle to overcome.

Transfiguration: A Mannequin Project

The papermaking project took place in an inpatient E.D. treatment program where I worked as an art therapist. Participants were predominantly White, cisgender females ranging in age from 12 to 66. The program was an acute level of care, with most patients admitted malnourished and underweight. Therefore, weight restoration was a crucial aspect of recovery. Processing the changes their bodies were undergoing and addressing body image were central themes. Art therapy was offered in a group setting. It occurred three times a week for 90 minutes.

After attending the Peace Paper Project workshop, I thought of using hand papermaking as a therapeutic way for patients to explore their body image and turn the clothes they had outgrown into empowering artwork. At the time I was also brainstorming ideas for an awareness art competition hosted by the International Association for Eating Disorder Professionals (I.A.E.D.P.) (http://www.iaedp.com). The annual event encouraged art therapists to collaborate with patients and decorate mannequins that reflected perceptions of beauty and healthy body image (Imagine Me, n.d.). My vision was to make paper from items of clothing that represented my clients' E.D.s and then sew the paper into a new garment for a size 16 mannequin, which is the clothing size of the average American woman (Christel & Dunn, 2017).

Session One

I began by presenting the idea to the patients and describing the process of making paper from clothing. We discussed the symbolism and significance of clothing and size labels in the context of body image distortion and E.D. recovery. Patients were encouraged to reflect on emotional attachments to items of clothing that represented their E.D. They explored what it would be like to let go of these garments and transform them into something more aligned with recovery and radical self-love. The group generated a list of intention words to guide the project: *energy, peace, health, strength, and love.*

Session Two

Patients brought personal items of clothing to repurpose into paper. As they cut the fabric into pieces, each shared the significance of their item and what it was like to cut it up. One patient chose a pair of jeans that held unfulfilled promises of "success, achievement, and self-confidence." Another chose a long underwear shirt she associated with being cold because of insufficient body fat.

I observed that, as they engaged in the repetitive and tactile activity of cutting the fabric, they spoke more openly and easily about their memories and associations. This was consistent with what other art therapists have observed about kinesthetic and sensory work in trauma treatment (Lusebrink & Hinz, 2016; Elbrecht, 2013). Specifically, it releases tension, awakens the senses, elicits pre-verbal bodily memories, and establishes healing rhythms. The cloth fragments were taken to Richard's studio and transformed into pulp using a **Hollander beater.**

Session Three

Working in a grassy area just outside the hospital, Richard, Bucciarelli, and I taught participants how to **pull** and **couch** sheets. Some participants expressed initial hesitation about getting wet or messy. However, these concerns dissipated once they dipped their hands into the **vats** of **slurry** and slowly lifted out the **mould** and **deckle,** gently **shaking** it from side to side and back and forth. These steps facilitated the interweaving of the fibers as the water drained out.

In the past decade, there has been increased interest in body-based therapy approaches that integrate art-making with bilateral stimulation for the treatment of trauma-related disorders (Tripp, 2016). With hand papermaking, the process of **sheet formation**, with embodied, rhythmic, bilateral movements and multi-sensory engagement, offered the patients a safe, alternative way to regulate their nervous systems and experience a sense of balance and integration. After couching the sheets, **pulp printing** was used with cardboard stencils to add the project's intention words: *energy, peace, health, strength, and love* (Figure 4.1).

Session Four

Patients drew images on the dried paper using oil pastels, representing their personal embodied experiences of the intention words. Processing the drawings, patients came to realize that their attempts to dissociate and numb their pain through E.D. behaviors had also limited their ability to feel pleasurable sensations and emotions.

Session Five

The group began with a discussion exploring the ways the body engages with the world through the senses to experience pleasure, connection, affection, and belonging. Patients were invited to write letters to their bodies expressing gratitude and appreciation. The letters were colored with markers, cut into long triangular strips, and rolled into colorful paper beads. The beads were strung together to create a necklace for the mannequin.

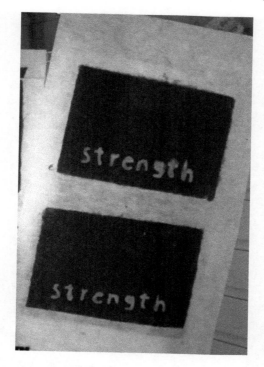

Figure 4.1 Intention words pulp printed on paper sheets.

Session Six

Off-site, Richard, Bucciarelli, and I sewed the group's paper together creating a dress for the mannequin. The completed mannequin was brought back to the hospital and put on display in the art therapy room (Figure 4.2). It was also submitted to the I.A.E.D.P. art competition. This final session with patients was spent processing the entire project. Themes of transformation, healing, growth, and radical self-love were discussed on individual, community, and societal levels. The patients marveled. Clothes that had symbolized so much shame and self-loathing had been transformed into something of which they felt proud.

Project Summary

Over several weeks of hand papermaking, patients at an eating disorder treatment center created new meaning from their experiences of restoring weight. Moreover, they developed a healthier relationship with their bodies. The embodied process of transforming skinny jeans into a plus-size party dress offered participants a paradigm shift – one in which radical self-love was possible.

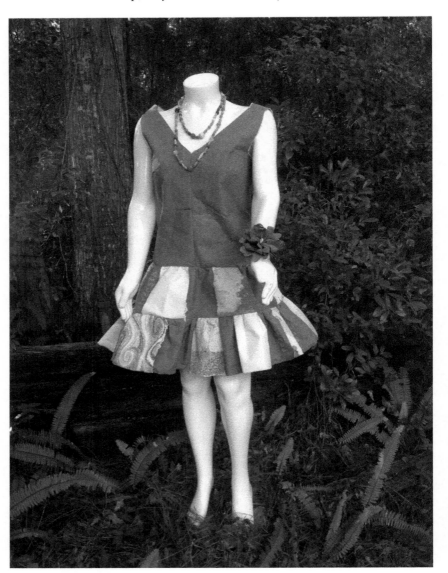

Figure 4.2 Transfiguration mannequin.

Hand Papermaking in Hospital-Based Medical Settings

Amy Bucciarelli

Medical hospitalization is a means to long-term healing and wellness; however, the experience can result in psychological concerns such as emotional distress, lost independence, social isolation, grief, and fear of death (Anand, 2016; Councill, 1999; Bucciarelli et al., 2020; David, 2016). Art therapists who are part of the multidisciplinary clinical team, support patients' psychosocial well-being during hospitalization (Bucciarelli, 2016; David, 2016). Malchiodi (1999) noted that in medical art therapy "the creative process of art-making focuses on something else besides the illness, disability, or dysfunction" (p. 17). Mastery of art materials and learning new artistic methods – like papermaking – can boost patients' self-esteem, confidence, sense of pleasure, and resilience (Councill, 2012). Additionally, art provides an outlet for expressing feelings related to illness, and the artwork becomes a tangible legacy memorializing the patient's experiences (Bucciarelli et al., 2020).

Inspired by the E.D. project, I wanted to make papermaking accessible to medical patients. With the help of Camp and Richard, I adapted the papermaking process for one-on-one work with patients at their hospital bedside. The patients, ages 5 to 21, were living with assistive medical devices while waiting for heart transplants. Due to medical needs, they were, by-and-large, unable to leave their rooms. Patients were hospitalized from one month up to one year, until they received their transplant – the timing of which was unknown. In an environment where most things were out of their control, hand papermaking empowered patients to **activate** the well parts of themselves, shift their identity, and transform their difficult situations into productive, meaningful experiences.

Adaptations for Medical Settings

Typically, papermaking is a multi-step process requiring specialized equipment, access to large amounts of water, and significant physical space (Heller, 1978), none of which are good in medical settings. Adapting the process required thoughtful attention to patients' energy levels, the safety of materials related to their medical conditions, and space constraints. Alternatives were devised for preparing and storing pulp, simplifying the papermaking process, and reducing the volume of water needed (Table 4.1).

Health Considerations

When choosing art media, infection precautions were important to consider, especially if patients were immunocompromised (Davis, 2021)[1]. Papermaking materials needed to be sanitized, individually packaged, or disposable.

Table 4.1 Adapted steps for hand papermaking at the hospital bedside

Papermaking Step	Adaptation	Description
Prepare the fibers	• Therapist/artist helps cut fabric	• Patients taking blood thinners may not be allowed to use scissors. Unsafe if they accidentally cut themselves.
Create the pulp	• Reconstitute desiccated dried/pressed pulp chips in a kitchen blender • Distilled water	• Blend 1 pulp chip with distilled water. Repeat until desired amount of pulp. • 1 chip of pulp (approx. 1 oz) yields 2 sheets of 5 × 8-inch paper.
Prepare the vat and couching surface	• 2 plastic containers with flat top lids used for vats • 1 piece of corrugated plastic sheeting for board • 2 synthetic shammies for bottom felts • 3–6 disposable non-fusible cloth interfacings for layering between paper sheets • 1 qt. bottle of distilled water	• All materials need to be smaller than the vat lids but larger than the paper. • Vat 1 for excess water. Vat 2 for pulling paper. • Vat lid 1 for sponging excess water before couching. Vat lid 2 as couching surface. • On vat lid 2, layer 1 corrugated pad, 1 shammie, 1 dampened interfacing. • Use water as needed to refresh vat 2.
Pull the paper	• Student-sized deckle box 5 × 8 inches • Reconstituted pulp in single-serving Tupperware (yellow-isolation masks; blue-gowns; white-sheets)	• Submerge deckle box in vat 2 with 1 inch of water. Pour pulp into deckle box and arrange with desired paper design. • Lift paper out of water. Remove top of deckle box and tilt to drain water into vat.
Couch the paper	• Piece of window screening slightly larger than paper • Kitchen sponge • Optional: poly-coated wooden block • Optional: pulp printing, pulp painting, and/or stenciling materials for embellishing paper design	• Place mould with paper on vat lid 1. • Lay screening over paper. • Gently press sponge into screen. Squeeze excess water into vat 1. • Peel screen off the paper. • Transfer paper onto vat 2 lid with layered couching materials. • Optional: slide block over mould screen before lifting. Allows paper to be easily released. Therapist/artist can offer hand-over-hand assistance if needed.
Dry the paper	• 3–4 plexiglass display stands 8½ × 11 inches (can use both sides for 8 total sheets of paper) • Large soft bristled flat paintbrush	• Lay sheet of paper on interfacing paper-side down on plexiglass. • Firmly brush backside of interfacing. • Peel interfacing off. Paper is tension-adhered to plexiglass. • Place plexiglass in safe space for paper to dry.

For example, corrugated plastic sheets that could be disinfected were used for couching boards. Bottom felts were synthetic shammies that could be laundered. Disposable, non-fusible cloth **interfacing** was used between sheets. Hospital gowns, sheets, and masks were laundered before being repurposed into pulp; they were donated by the hospital because they were ripped or frayed.

In other papermaking workshops, fibers were pulped in large batches and stored for future use in tubs with water. This situation can result in bacterial growth. Needing a hygienic method for hospital work, I learned I could **press** and **dry** pulp into dehydrated **"pulp chips,"** which could be stored in individual plastic bags and reconstituted in a blender with distilled water. This innovation allowed me to prepare small on-demand batches of pulp for individual patients.

Frequently, hospitalized patients have low energy and attention for artistic processes due to their medical conditions (Bucciarelli, 2019). On average, these patients had the stamina to make 3–6 sheets of paper per session. Along the way, I discovered helpful adaptive tricks. For instance, patients often lacked hand-arm strength to press the paper into the interfacing when couching: sliding a poly-coated block of wood across the back of the **deckle box** screen amplified pressure, allowing the paper to release.

Simplifying the papermaking process

Art-making in medical settings has logistical challenges (Bucciarelli, 2019; David, 2016). Sessions done on small bedside tables offer limited space. To address this issue, I used a rolling cart to store and transport materials, so papermaking was both modular and mobile (Figure 4.3). Patients could sit at the edge of the bed, using the cart as a working surface (Figure 4.4). If we were interrupted for medical consultations or treatments, I could easily and quickly roll the cart out of the room.

A major modification I had to make was reducing the amount of water and controlling its extraction. Deckle boxes, instead of **European-style moulds and deckles**, required less water in the vat. It still allowed the patient to pour and arrange pulp across the mould within a thin layer of water. Once formed, the sheet was drained normally. Before couching, a screen was placed over the paper to protect it, while excess water was sponged from the sheet. After the patient couched the paper, additional water was removed in this manner.

A final adaptation was **restraint drying** the sheets on plexiglass display stands just larger than the pressed paper. The paper was easily transferred from the interfacing to the plexiglass by using a large paintbrush to smooth over the back of the interfacing, adhering the paper to the plexiglass. The plexi-stands were placed in hospital room corners or windowsills while the paper dried. It was therapeutically important for patients to keep the paper in their possession. This underscored their active participation in a process of transformation from start to finish. It was also fun to watch the paper dry!

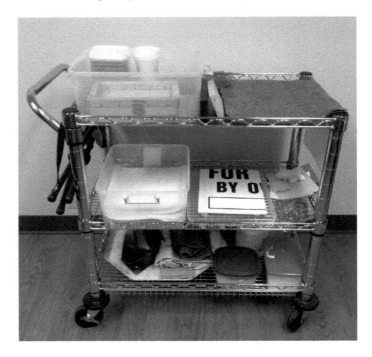

Figure 4.3 Cart with supplies for hospital bedside papermaking.

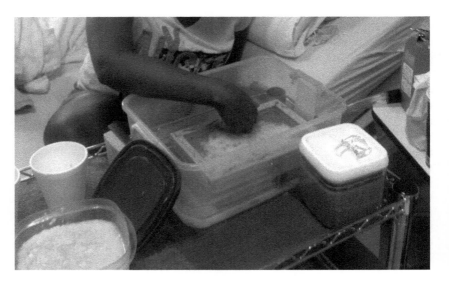

Figure 4.4 Patient making paper at the bedside.

Symbolism of Hand Papermaking for Heart Transplant Patients

Identity

The patients who made paper were independent, healthy young people who suddenly became medically dependent. Overnight, their identity changed. Tina Mullin, director of the U.F. Health Shands Arts in Medicine (https://artsinmedicine.ufhealth.org) program, described the inherently depersonalizing experience of being admitted to a hospital:

The first thing that happens is they remove your personal belongings. Your clothes [a part of your personal expression and identity] are taken away from you. You are given a hospital gown to wear, and your clothes are handed back to your loved one in a plastic bag. You no longer make choices about what to wear or even who enters your hospital room. The most basic choices are no longer under your control. Often, you are identified by your medical record number or your diagnosis: "patient with Osteosarcoma in room 245B."

(personal communication, September 17, 2021)

Medical garments represented the social and emotional dehumanization of the patient experience. Breaking them down to make paper mirrored a deconstruction/reconstruction of the patient's own identity – person to patient, then to artist. It also served as a cathartic release of the frustrations, grief, and fears that accompany hospitalization. Through the papermaking process, the fibers were reimagined. The patient has a sense of control by choosing the new "identity" of the fibers; they may be formed into paper for a card to a caregiver, part of a journal for writing intimate thoughts, or a work of art proudly displayed in their room.

Death-Rebirth

Patients with significant medical conditions have conscious or unconscious awareness that they are living within the liminal space of life and death (Anand, 2016; Council, 2012; Malchiodi, 1999). As easily as a hallmate can leave the hospital with a clean bill of health, someone in the next room could unexpectedly die. The cycle of life – birth, death, and rebirth – becomes an important symbolic theme in medical art therapy. Patients were acutely aware of their lifecycle and their earthly existence. During treatment, hospitalized patients also experience many other "lifecycles" of transformation. For example, the cycle of a round of medication or chemotherapy.

Heart transplant patients especially are close to the death-rebirth experience. A donor must *die* so that the heart transplant patient can receive a new heart and *live*. Hoping for a successful transplant, they are wheeled to surgery and drift into anesthesia-induced sleep, a "death" to their old self. When they wake up from the procedure, they are physically changed. They have a new heart and a renewed sense of life. It is in fact a rebirth.

Hand papermaking becomes a relevant parallel process for the death-rebirth narratives that accompany hospitalization. The recycled fabric turns elemental as it is beaten into a pulp, becoming part of the watery slurry in preparation for papermaking. As pulp, the substance *is* potentiality. It died from its old form; now it is full of possibilities, waiting for rebirth. Reconstituted pulp is poured into the deckle box and submerged in water. The patient's hands sculpt the pulp into something new, the fibers are reformed. The sheet of paper is pulled out of the water, alchemically revived – birthed anew. Fibers once associated with "sickness" and "hospitalization," gain new life as creative masterpieces, as beautiful sheets of paper.

Project Summary

Adapting the papermaking for hospitalized patients challenged me to break down each step of the papermaking process and discover how to make it simple, portable, and modular. Safety and space constraints required creative innovation. Ultimately, patients enjoyed the artistic process, which was embedded with therapeutic metaphors about life.

Hand Papermaking with Students with Learning Disabilities

Amy Koski Richard

After meaningful collaborations with the Peace Paper Project and art therapists Bucciarelli and Camp, I continued connecting with different populations through papermaking. Part of this journey involved a series of Artist in Residence projects with Arts4All Florida (https://www.arts4allflorida.org), a program dedicated to supporting arts education and cultural experiences for and by people with disabilities (Arts4All Florida, 2019). The program pairs teaching artists with Exceptional Student Education (E.S.E.) teachers who are seeking creative experiences for their students. Artists were encouraged to teach their chosen art form, an ideal way to expand my papermaking horizons.

I was matched with several elementary and middle schools in rural communities where I collaborated with teachers and their students. The students ranged from kindergarten to ninth grade. The students represented a range of disabilities that impact learning including, autism spectrum disorders, muscular dystrophy, attention deficit hyperactivity disorder, and oppositional defiant disorder. Some students lacked basic learning skills such as reading, writing, or speaking.

Higher functioning students struggled with "hidden" gaps in their abilities while demonstrating above-average intelligence. Others were identified for E.S.E. due to behavioral issues. Many of the disabilities were the result of genetic and/or neurobiological factors that interfered with learning capabilities, and other cognitive skills, such as organization, memory, attention span, or reasoning (Learning Disabilities Association of America, n.d.). These challenges translated into struggles with coping and basic life skills at home and school.

Adapting to a Classroom Environment

The main challenge with portable papermaking was water management. Easy access to water and containing it while working was the key to portable papermaking. A common solution was to work outside; however, this was not always feasible due to disrupting other classes or discipline challenges. Time constraints were a further issue. Each residency needed 90 minutes to two hours. Therefore, the process, including setup, breakdown, and repacking for another school on the same day, needed streamlining (Figure 4.5).

As in hospital settings, one strategy that reduced the need for water was working with deckle boxes that required much less water. Deckle boxes had other advantages: a) they provided an ideal informal assessment tool for gauging hand skills and overall abilities such as measuring and pouring water and pulp; b) one could manipulate the pulp inside the box; and c) one could lock/unlock the mould

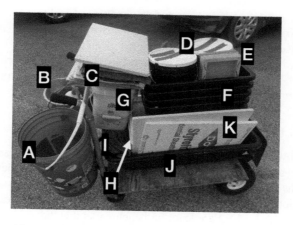

Figure 4.5 Portable papermaking cart for the classroom.

A) 5-gallon bucket for multi-purpose; B) 2-gallon bucket with several 1-gallon buckets nested inside for multi-use; C) 20 to 30 cloth interfacing felts; D) 2-gallon buckets with prepared pulp; E) 2 to 4 deckle boxes/moulds and deckles; F) 2-gallon buckets with prepared pulp; G) 3-gallon bucket with holes drilled for straining; H) 4 shallow couching trays (24 × 18 × 3 inches); I) 8 to 10 wool felts for bottom/top of posts; J) 1 large plastic vat for "catch-all"; K) half-inch foam insulation boars for couching.

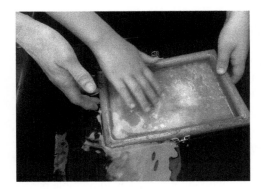

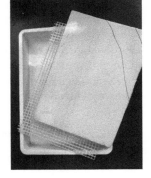

Figure 4.6 Deckle box.   *Figure 4.7* Couching tray.

after sheet-forming. Students in grades 3 to 5 used 5.5 × 8-inch moulds for easier handling, while older students used a larger 8.5 × 11-inch size. As I learned from Bucciarelli and Camp, the deckle box also provided physical and metaphoric "containment" (Lusebrink & Hinz, 2016). It served as a boundary for students with behavior challenges and a holding vessel for those overwhelmed by large amounts of water and pulp (Figure 4.6).

The most important logistical modification was developing a couching system for capturing excess water (Figure 4.7). Using couching sheets on lightweight foam insulation boards with felts, positioned inside 3-inch-deep trays, allowed us to pour off excess water as needed, without disturbing the sheets. In addition, these trays were used to transport freshly made sheets to my studio to be de-watered in a hydraulic press and dried in a "stack dryer", providing high-quality paper. The students' excitement about receiving their artwork at the next session was an added benefit.

Curriculum Development

Teachers know that organization and preparation are keys to success in the classroom. For an artist accustomed to less formal workshop formats, developing lesson plans was an adjustment. A related challenge was aligning the activities with state education standards. In Florida, Collaborate, Plan, Align, Learn, Motivate and Share (C.P.A.L.M.S.) are learning benchmarks that "identify what students are expected to know or do as a result of what they learn in class" for each grade level (Florida Education Foundation, 1984, para. 1). These standards include color and shape recognition and increasing vocabulary, along with specific math skills and science concepts. Daunting at first, this practice grew easier as I became familiar with the standards and began identifying aspects of papermaking that were relevant to science, language arts, visual arts, and life skills (Table 4.2).

Table 4.2 Curricular-based projects for classroom hand papermaking with E.S.E. students

Project Descriptions	Learning Benchmarks (Fourth-grade examples)
Project 1 – Cloud Paper This first activity allows assessment of abilities for future adaptations; often combined with Project 2. **Discussion:** Clouds, rain, weather, etc. **Activity:** Students mix blue (pigmented) cotton or **abaca** pulp and water into small 32 oz. containers before pouring into the deckle box and repeating this same step with while cotton pulp (i.e., the clouds).	**Visual Arts:** Experiment with various materials, tools, techniques, and processes to achieve a variety of results in two- and/or three-dimensional artworks. **Visual Arts:** Follow procedures for using tools, media, techniques, and processes safely and responsibly. **Earth and Space Science:** Compare and describe changing patterns in nature that repeat themselves, such as weather conditions (including temperature and precipitation), day-to-day, and season-to-season.
Project 2 – Old fashioned paper Coined by a fourth grader who was thrilled by the spontaneous marbling effect, harkening to the "days of old." **Discussion:** Introduces concept of paper made from **cellulose** fibers (cotton and hemp). **Activity:** Reinforcing steps learned from cloud paper, students measure cotton pulp and water and pour slurry into the deckle box, followed by hemp pulp. The slurry is then mixed with students' hands inside the deckle box to achieve a marbling effect.	**Visual Arts:** Integrate the structural elements of art and organizational principles of design with sequential procedures and techniques to achieve an artistic goal. **Visual Arts:** Develop craftsmanship skills through repeated practice. **Visual Arts:** Demonstrate the ability to recall art procedures and focus on art processes through to the end of production.
Project 3 – Seed paper Supports classroom curricula about plants and reproductive processes. Sequential steps and cooperation are reinforced by helping one another follow detailed instructions. **Discussion:** Paper can be made in different shapes; seeds can be embedded into handmade paper, dried, and later planted in dirt so the seeds can sprout into plants. **Activity:** Students mix specific amounts of water and pulp before adding seeds and then pouring into D.I.Y. plastic circular "deckle boxes," draining and then couching onto tray.	**Science:** Distinguish plants based on common and scientific names. **Science:** Compare and contrast major stages in the life cycles of Florida plants and animals, such as those that undergo incomplete and complete metamorphosis, and flowering and non-flowering seed-bearing plants. **Science:** Identify processes of sexual reproduction in flowering plants, including pollination, fertilization (seed production), seed dispersal, and germination.

(Continued)

Table 4.2 (Continued)

Project Descriptions	Learning Benchmarks (Fourth-grade examples)
Project 4 – Nature Print Paper Provides students an opportunity to study and observe forms in nature. **Discussion:** Students show and discuss plants they collected, their names, and the diversity of shapes and forms found in the leaves, fruits, stems, etc. **Activity:** European and/or **Nepalese-style** sheet formation followed by pulp printing using leaves, ferns and other natural objects as "stencils."	**Visual Arts:** Identify the structural elements of art used to unite an artistic composition. **Science:** Distinguish plants based on common and scientific names. **Science:** Although characteristics of plants and animals are inherited, some characteristics can be affected by the environment.
Project 5 – Expressive Paper Reinforcing new skills, students practice sequential directions with new opportunities for self-expression. **Discussion:** Students listen to and discuss music and how different kinds make them feel [loud, fast, slow, relaxing, exciting]. **Activity:** Sheets formed using floating moulds; pulp "paint" used to make expressive lines while listening to music. Squeeze bottles of pigmented pulp are traded between students when music changes to allow use of multiple colors.	**Communication** – Perform: solidify group cohesion toward an assigned task using both verbal and non-verbal skills. **Music:** Examine and explain how expressive elements, when used in a selected musical work, affect personal response. **Visual Arts:** Demonstrate the ability to recall art procedures and focus on art processes through to the end of production.
Project 6 – European-style Papermaking and Pulp Printing Students comfortable with the papermaking process made paper using European-style mould and deckles and vat with water and pulp. **Discussion:** Introduce history of European papermaking and concept of paper made from rags that are fermented (retted) to process into pulp. **Activity:** After forming sheets students make imagery using stencils and pulp printing techniques.	**Visual Arts:** Through purposeful practice, artists learn to manage, master, and refine simple, then complex, skills and techniques. **Visual Arts:** Use accurate art vocabulary to discuss works of art and the creative process. **Visual Arts:** Follow procedures for using tools, media, techniques, and processes safely and responsibly. **Science:** Identify familiar changes in materials that result in materials with different characteristics, such as decaying animal or plant matter, burning, rusting, and cooking.

(Continued)

Table 4.2 (Continued)

Project Descriptions	Learning Benchmarks (Fourth-grade examples)
Project 7 – Watermarks Adapting historical watermark techniques, students make paper with "invisible" imagery made visible when backlit. **Discussion:** Students identify favorite animals and explore ideas of spirit animals from American Indian culture. **Activity:** Students trace simple line drawings of spirit animals onto open-weave cloth and then re-trace with puffy paint to prepare for making watermark. The cloth is used on top of the mould when sheet-forming, resulting in a watermark in the handmade sheet.	**Visual Arts:** Through study in the arts, we learn about and honor others and the worlds in which they live(d). **Visual Arts:** The arts reflect and document cultural trends and historical events and help explain how new directions in the arts have emerged. **Science:** Manipulate lighting effects, using various media to create desired results.

With each residency, repetition and experience led to curricular improvements. For example, printed step-by-step instructions for sheet formation reinforced sequential learning. The added benefit was it provided clear instructions for teachers and assistants, most of whom were experiencing papermaking for the first time. Additional strategies included numbering the tools and materials and arranging them in sequence. This inspired games when students began counting the steps together and correcting one another, spontaneously building cooperation.

To target goals identified by the teachers, papermaking activities were tailored to cultivate focus and skill-building while fostering creativity and cooperation among students (Table 4.3). Small, but meaningful successes were observed. In one instance, a student took it upon herself to mentor a classmate who was prone to impulsive acts like emptying buckets of water on the floor. With patience beyond her years, I watched in amazement as she assisted her classmate in making paper. Others encouraged classmates who were reluctant to try the process, often with more success than the adults who tried to encourage the students.

Table 4.3 Common goals for classroom hand papermaking with ESE students

- Increase accessibility to art
- Increase one-on-one instruction
- Reinforce cooperation among students
- Strengthen coordination and hand skills, including fine and gross motor skills
- Cultivate focus
- Reinforce life skills (e.g., following sequential instructions, coping and communication skills, creative and critical thinking, decision-making, interpersonal skills, problem-solving, self-awareness, self-soothing, and stress management

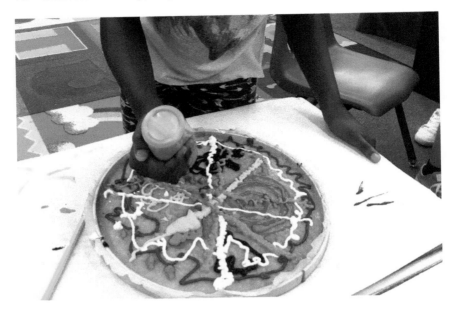

Figure 4.8 Expressive circle paper.

Keeping students excited about new techniques while reinforcing learned skills was important and sometimes led to discoveries. Experiments with circular floating moulds made with needlepoint hoops and crinoline cloth screens paired beautifully with pulp writing techniques using finely beaten pulp applied through a squeeze bottle (Figure 4.8). Simultaneously, this was a solution for sensory-averse students who were uncomfortable getting water or pulp on their hands. This adaptation helped increase their expressiveness. The artwork could remain in the classroom because the paper stayed on the mould without pressing. This allowed the students to watch their paper change over time as it dried, a science observation benchmark.

At the end of each residency, success was measured by students' abilities to complete the projects along with on-site evaluations. One of the evaluations completed by an E.S.E. teacher estimated that 75–100% of her students achieved an increase in: artistic skills; self-expression; cooperation and communication, including new vocabulary terms; creative thinking; improvement in fine and gross motor skills; willingness to try new things; and following directions. Improved behavior, communication skills, and increased retention of information were observed among 50–74% of students. One teacher identified "critical and creative thinking and willingness to try new things" as students' top growth areas from the papermaking residency (personal communication, May 20, 2019).

Project Summary

Engaging with the Arts4All training resources for working with special needs students was crucial to the residency's success. Pre-planning meetings with teachers provided opportunities for discussing students' abilities, challenges, and classroom dynamics before each residency. Modifying the labor-intensive papermaking process to be portable and sustainable for the teaching artist was also critical.

Observing the students and letting them inform the process was equally important. For example, it was evident setting up was as valuable as making paper. This created anticipation and rituals that were repeated with each visit. Filling vats, preparing pulp, arranging couching boards, and wetting felts and pressing them with a rolling pin, helped everyone relax, center, and focus.

The enthusiasm of the teachers and assistants as they joined their students in making paper was a reminder that art is important for all of us, regardless of age and ability. Despite all the triumphs, the most difficult aspect of this work was saying goodbye at the end of each residency. As I worked with the class for numerous sessions, a sense of familiarity developed as students eagerly prepared for each papermaking session. Years later, I still remember their sweet faces.

Conclusions

Like a pebble dropped into water, the ripples created from these unexpected connections have traveled greater distances than we could have imagined, catalyzing many defining moments. Like any collaboration, opportunities for learning move in multiple directions. Thanks to the knowledge of art therapists, an artist was able to articulate the therapeutic benefits of papermaking experienced in the studio while also discovering new ways of adapting the practice for others in the community. In return, art therapists gained meaningful technical expertise and guidance for bringing this practice to healthcare populations and colleagues, widening the circle even more.

Note

1 This project took place prior to the COVID-19 pandemic. Infection control guidelines differ between healthcare systems and should be considered for papermaking projects in medical settings.

References

American Psychiatric Association. (2013). *Diagnostic and statistical manual of mental disorders* (5th ed.). American Psychiatric Publishing.

Anand, S. A. (2016). Dimensions of art therapy in medical illness. In D. Gussak & M. Rosal (Eds.), *The Wiley handbook of art therapy* (pp. 409–420). Wiley Blackwell.

Arts4All Florida. (2019). Home. https://www.arts4allflorida.org.

Bucciarelli, A. (2016). The art therapies: Approaches, goals, and integration in arts in health. In S. Clift & P. Camic (Eds.), *Oxford textbook of creative arts, health, and wellbeing* (pp. 271–279). Oxford University.

Bucciarelli, A. (2019). Utilizing tablet computers in art therapy for young people with chronic and life-limiting illnesses. In M. Wood, B. Jacobson, & H. Cridford (Eds.), *The international handbook of art therapy in palliative and bereavement care* (pp. 110–125). Routledge.

Bucciarelli, A., Ellison, G., Sommer, E., & Spooner, H. (2020). The arts in health settings. In W. IsHak (Ed.), *The handbook of wellness medicine* (pp. 454–466). Cambridge University.

Christel, D. A. & Dunn. S. C. (2017). Average American women's clothing size: Comparing National Health and Nutritional Examination Surveys (1988–2010) to ASTM International Misses & Women's Plus Size clothing. *International Journal of Fashion Design, Technology, and Education, 10*(2), 129–136. https://doi.org/10.1080/17543266. 2016.1214291.

Costin, C. (2007). *The eating disorder sourcebook* (3rd ed.). McGraw-Hill.

Councill, T. (1999). Art therapy with pediatric cancer patients. In. C. Malchiodi (Ed.), *Medical art therapy with children* (pp. 75–93). Jessica Kingsley Publishers.

Councill, T. (2012) Medical art therapy with children. In C. Malchiodi (Ed.), *Handbook of art therapy* (2nd ed.) (pp. 222–240). Guilford Press.

David, I. R. (2016). Art therapy in medical settings. In D. Gussak & M. Rosal (Eds.), *The Wiley handbook of art therapy* (pp. 443–450). Wiley Blackwell.

Davis, A. (2021). Infection control and art supplies: The tools of our trade. In M. Itczak (Ed.), *Pediatric medical art therapy* (pp. 25–37). Jessica Kingsley Publishers.

Elbrecht, C. (2013). *Trauma and healing at the clay field: A sensorimotor art therapy approach*. Jessica Kingsley Publishers.

Florida Education Foundation. (1984). K12 Florida Standards. https://www.cpalms.org/CPALMS/about_us.aspx.

Heller, J. (1978). *Papermaking*. Watson-Guptill.

Imagine Me (n.d.) International Association for Eating Disorder Professionals Foundation. http://www.iaedp.com/imagine-me.

King, J. L. (Ed.). (2016). *Art therapy, trauma, and neuroscience: Theoretical and practical perspectives*. Routledge.

Learning Disabilities Association of America. (n.d.). Types of learning disabilities. https://ldaamerica.org/types-of-learning-disabilities.

Lusebrink, V. B., & Hinz, L. D. (2016). The expressive therapies continuum as a framework in the treatment of trauma. In J. L. King (Ed.), *Art therapy, trauma and neuroscience: Theoretical and practical perspectives* (pp. 42–66). Routledge.

Malchiodi, C. (1999). Introduction to medical art therapy with children. In. C. Malchiodi (Ed.), *Medical art therapy with children* (pp.13–32). Jessica Kingsley Publishers.

Peace Paper Project (n.d.). Home. Peace Paper Project. http://www.peacepaperproject.org.

Scatoloni, P. (2019). Somatic experiencing: The body as the missing link in eating disorder treatment. In A. Seubert & P. Verdi (Eds.), *Trauma-informed approaches to eating disorders* (pp. 275–285). Springer.

Seubert, A. J., & Virdi, P. (2019). *Trauma-informed approaches to eating disorders*. Springer.

Strings, S. (2019). *Fearing the black body: The racial origins of fat phobia.* New York University.

Taylor, S. R. (2018). *The body is not an apology: The power of radical self-love.* Berrett-Koehler.

Tripp, T. (2016). A body-based bilateral art protocol for reprocessing trauma. In J. L. King (Ed.), *Art therapy, trauma and neuroscience: Theoretical and practical perspectives* (pp. 174–194). Routledge.

5 Papermaking Transformation in an Art Therapy Curriculum

Janice M. Havlena

From a weekend workshop for students with the Peace Paper Project to the creation of on-site and portable papermaking studio projects, this chapter follows the journey of an undergraduate art therapy program and its community outreach across age, culture, and abilities. Along the way art therapy students develop skills in papermaking and an appreciation for how it can give voice to youth, older adults, people living with epilepsy, and self-taught artists with disabilities, as well as an enhancement of their own art practice.

About Undergraduate Art Therapy

The purpose and content of undergraduate art therapy education are not the same as for the graduate-level student. A master's degree is required for entry-level practice in art therapy: undergraduate studies in art therapy do not lead to professional art therapist credentials. However, undergraduate art therapy educators, Schwartz et al. (2021), have acknowledged the contributions of bachelor's level art therapy education in generating interest in the field and preparing students for graduate work. Their study of art therapy undergraduate programs found curricula ranging from a single course to concentrations, minors, and majors. Likewise, the goals of those offerings varied from introduction to the field to graduate school preparation.

Requirements of art studio courses were typically classes necessary as prerequisites by most graduate art therapy programs. Historically, art therapy pioneer, Edith Kramer, encouraged serious art practice for art therapists (Kramer & Gerity, 2000). Moon (2001) advanced the need for cultivating an artist's identity. Allen (1992) emphasized the importance of art practice in student training. Schwartz et al. (2021) reasoned those undergraduate art therapy curricula with more art studio requirements "may eventually yield professional art therapists who have an enhanced artist-identity and wider knowledge of materials" (p. 6).

DOI: 10.4324/9781003216261-8

Edgewood College's Undergraduate Art Therapy Major

Within the art department at Edgewood College (http://www.edgewoodcollege.edu), the undergraduate art therapy major was designed to introduce students to the field of art therapy, develop their knowledge and skills in community art programs, and cultivate their abilities and commitment to their growth as artists. Preparation for graduate school also guided the curriculum. Major requirements included art therapy and psychology courses, studio art, art history, practicum, and internship. In addition, students were required to develop a formal art portfolio and presentation.

The Papermaking Proposal

The art therapy program was an established major when I proposed papermaking as an addition to the curriculum. During this time, founding members of the Peace Paper Project were conducting a two-day workshop on papermaking and trauma therapy on campus. They opened with an evening lecture about their history, mission, and work. Over the next two days, art therapy students rotated through sessions on **rag** preparation, sheet production, creative writing, and art therapy applications of papermaking. The workshop fueled unprecedented interest, engagement, and productivity, demonstrating how papermaking could support community art, student development, and curriculum goals.

A new art and theater building was at a pre-blueprint stage; therefore, it could include space for papermaking. The new building presented a possible opening to grow this medium. Seizing the opportunity to consult with Drew Matott, I rolled out the architects' drawings. Matott suggested key, non-structural modifications that would allow the new, projected "mixed media" studio classroom to function more effectively as a dedicated papermaking studio. He and I continued to work together to plan and create this space (DeLamater, 2016). Matott also shared resources for equipment, tools, supplies, materials, and additional areas to study.

Papermaking was a good fit with the mission of the art therapy program. Papermaking had the potential to advance the program's emphasis on community art initiatives. It would also strengthen partnerships by hosting papermaking experiences on- and off-campus. Papermaking was consistent with the department's goals because it was an inherently green art medium, and it used low-tech equipment that could be used wherever needed.

Internal college funding sources were sought to support the papermaking proposal. These resources were leveraged for equipment, supplies, and faculty development. For example, I attended a week-long in-residence, intensive course in papermaking. Consultation with the Peace Paper Project assisted with the setup and training on the new equipment. The launch of the papermaking studio coincided with the opening of the new building in Fall 2012. The Peace Paper Project's scheduled tour also permitted Matott to create and teach a studio art papermaking course for the spring semester. As of this writing, adjunct studio art faculty continue to teach this course, which has remained open to all students.

Transformation of the Curriculum

Papermaking Coursework

To integrate papermaking into the art therapy major, I developed multiple units of study across several courses. In the pre-practicum art media and methods course, student-led teams designed, demonstrated, and facilitated on-campus workshops for selected community partners. One of the teams, along with a small group of visitors, would create and lead a papermaking process during class. In the Community Art Practicum, the entire class was taught papermaking skills over several weeks. In addition, the class planned and conducted a Fall semester, off-campus, public workshop. Similarly, as seniors, students had an opportunity to implement papermaking at their art therapy internship sites. Students also had the option to pursue advanced skills in the papermaking art studio course, some creating work they included in their senior art portfolios.

Workshop Formats

On-Campus Workshops

One- and two-day workshops took place on-site in the papermaking studio. The space could accommodate up to 24 participants over two days. On day one, the group engaged in making paper. On day two, participants worked with their handmade papers to create art with media such as, but not limited to, drawing, printmaking, collage, bookmaking, and creative writing. One-day workshops were an option for participants to engage in making paper in the on-campus studio. Art therapy students would work with participants at their site to cut rag that would then be **pulped** on campus. Once it was dried, the paper would then be returned to the community partner's site. When the paper was returned, the students also led a discussion and a reflection with the group about the process.

Off-Campus Workshops

These workshops were led by students at community partner sites. The format incorporated many of the same processes mentioned previously for on-campus sessions. Options for **pressing** and **drying** the paper included the following: a) the human press method and window **restraint drying** at the site; or b) returning the sheets to the papermaking studio to press and dry.

Public Outdoor Workshops

This format used kiosk posters and displays to orient drop-in participants to the workshop purpose and process. A portable **Oracle beater** was used primarily for these outdoor demonstrations. The human press method served as an effective way to involve participants in pressing the paper and was easy to transport. Pre-made handmade papers created by students were also stacked for participants to "make and take." Students prepared lightweight rigid surfaces from recycled materials so participants could safely save their paper and take it home.

The Papermaking Studio

Located next door to the art therapy classroom, the papermaking studio included adjacent offices, storage, display, and gathering spaces. The studio featured a separate beater room with a floor sink, ventilation, locking cabinets, large utility sinks, stainless steel counters with electrical outlets, a fume hood, and open shelving for supplies and student work. A digital teaching station, whiteboard, adjustable tables, and stackable chairs supported lectures and presentations (Figure 5.1).

Initially, the papermaking studio was equipped with a portable Oracle beater, utility cart, hydraulic jack **press** with an angle-iron frame mounted on a rolling platform, and a large-format, stacking restraint dryer with box fans and plastic sheet cover for controlled drying. A few years later, a 2-lb. **Reina beater** and tabletop hydraulic jack press were purchased with internal grant funds.

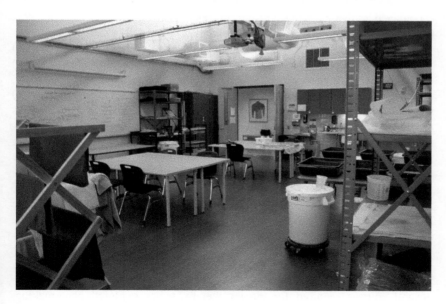

Figure 5.1 Papermaking studio. Photo by Robert Tarrell.

Classroom sets of 9 × 12, and 12 × 18-inch hardwood **moulds** and **deckles** and several sizes of **Nepalese-style moulds** made by Matott were used for classes and workshops. Composite poly utility mixing tubs served as portable **vats**. Accessories included paint strainers, **Pellon®**, wool felt blankets, plywood **post** boards, and assorted tools and supplies. Restraint drying was possible on the windows of the classroom, the adjacent hallway, and gathering spaces.

Papermaking Media Properties and Methods

Media Properties

Understanding the inherent characteristics of art media, and how an art process might be constructed, was essential for planning an effective process. One way media can be considered is by its resistive and fluid properties. For example, how wet and potentially uncontrolled it can be, or how dry and rigid a particular medium was experienced. Additionally, some media possessed both fluid and resistive properties (Malchiodi, 2011). These properties may also be mediated using tools or desirable quantities to adjust the user's control and experience (Hinz, 2016). Standard media used in art therapy have been paints, pastels, clay, and collage, but art therapists also use a variety of other media. Although Kramer (Ainlay Anand & Gerity, 2018) discouraged using "novel" media because it distracted from artistic production, Moon (2010) explored how "non-traditional" material can be appropriate and effective in contemporary practice. Likewise, Hinz (2016), encouraged art therapists to study and contribute their findings on different media to advance understanding of how art materials may be used in therapy.

Papermaking as a therapeutic medium presents unusual characteristics: a) while a novel process for many, paper itself is a common, familiar material; b) the art of hand papermaking has a long tradition and the idea of creating actual, usable handmade paper from beaten plant fiber appeals to the imagination; c) working with vats of paper **pulp** is a fluid process, yet the moulds and deckles provide structure. These tools can all be scaled to adjust user control. The multiple steps in the process, such as **charging the vat, pulling** a sheet, waiting for the mould to drain, **couching**, pressing, and drying, gradually distance the papermaker from the formless, wet pulp, and allow for observation and reflection. Also, like clay – a relatively fluid medium recognized for its therapeutic ability to be reworked (Fenner, 2016) – paper pulp and handmade papers can be rehydrated and re-pulped. Potentially, this can dispel fears of mistakes, failure, or wasting media – barriers that can inhibit creative experimentation.

Methods

Several courses required for the art therapy major explored papermaking. Other courses investigated a variety of art media and methods students might encounter and implement in community art program settings. When constructing art-making processes for participants, basic skills, safety, developmental stages in art, accessibility, and cultural identity were considered. Papermaking workshops with community partners tailored goals, materials, and types of processes to the unique visitor group and length of the session.

All workshops – on- and off-campus – incorporated some of the following features.

- **Equipment.** A **Hollander beater**, paper press, and restraint dryer were available.
- **Tools.** Moulds and deckles (9 × 12-inch were easier for beginners to use), vats and buckets for pulp, post boards, Pellon®, felts, sponges, plastic or wooden utensils for shaping, pencils, and strips of paper for labeling, small plastic containers, and scoopers.
- **Media.** Two or more colors of 100% cotton rag pulp from T-shirts or denim, selected **inclusions** such as, but not limited to, dried plant material, handmade or recycled paper scraps, natural materials, ribbons, or twine.
- **Set-up.** Several stations were arranged, each with a vat, bucket of pulp, moulds, deckles, inclusions, post boards, and tools. Tables were set up so they could be accessed from both sides. One or two art therapy students and one to three participants could be at each station.
- **Overview.** Orientation to hand papermaking included examples of plant fibers and handmade papers. Demonstration of the beater, introduction to moulds and deckles, pressing methods, and restraint drying were also provided.
- **Techniques.** A variety of techniques were introduced: a) ways to pull a **uniform sheet**; b) creating sheets with "**papermaker tears**"; c) using one hand on the mould as a stencil; d) couching; e) **double couching** with two colors; f) use of stencils to pull a formed shape; g) adding inclusions to the vat; and h) adding decorative material after pulling a sheet. Participant names were penciled on paper strips to label each sheet.
- **Themes.** Prompts ranged from suggestions for exploring the media and papermaking process to relevant topics and themes for the group of participants. These included pre-made examples of the completed work.
- **Reflection.** This included the group viewing the work and reacting to the papermaking process before pressing. The viewing, discussion, or journal writing about dried work and completed projects also took place.

Transformations with Community Partnerships

The art therapy curriculum emphasized and depended upon the community. It required initiating, developing, and sustaining partnerships. Both art and art therapy educators recognized the importance and power of art programming constructed in collaboration with communities. For example, Eça and Mason (2008) acknowledged the impact of art therapy programs on young people when programs were developed with "consideration of community and the goal of social justice" (p.14). We learned that experiences where college students engaged with these programs played an invaluable role in developing relationships between college students and community participants. They also tested and expanded students' ideas about their practice and their understanding of the individual communities (Timm-Bottos & Reilly, 2015).

Beginning with students' first experiences as facilitators during on-campus workshops, papermaking had been offered to visiting community partners. As they advanced, art therapy students worked in the community at a wide variety of sites. Students were challenged to support, cooperate, collaborate, and learn to assist with art projects, classes, and programs, and to offer creative art experiences, including papermaking, where none existed previously.

Observations

Papermaking consistently engaged individuals from a wide range of groups, backgrounds, and ages. Many of the positive outcomes students and community partners observed appeared to be inherent in the papermaking process itself. A sense of belonging developed among participants by sharing this process with others. Working cooperatively to cut rag, take turns, and share equipment, tools, materials, and space contributed to group cohesion. For example, assisting a peer in pulling and couching sheets, volunteering to walk on the human press, and stacking the **dry box** helped participants to feel valued. In addition, participants watched, assisted, and gathered ideas from others, which encouraged individuals to try the process at their own pace. The collaborative processes and flexibility of the pulp allowed individuals to develop the freedom to experiment and appreciate unexpected outcomes.

Partners

Adult Artists with Disabilities

ArtWorking (http://www.artworking.org), a Madison, Wisconsin, area non-profit program, provided career development and support for artists and entrepreneurs with disabilities. ArtWorking artists had been visitors to the art therapy student media workshops for many years prior to the addition of the papermaking studio. As a result, students learned about the artists, their artwork, creative processes, and how self-expression supported their well-being. Conversely, the artists were stimulated by working in a college studio alongside students, reinforcing their artist identity. Introduction to papermaking expanded the range of media the adult artists explored. Although many of the artists had strong preferences for art media and processes, most were interested in trying out the medium and they accepted the challenge to incorporate their own handmade papers artistically.

Adolescents

Almost all the teens from area youth programs were enthralled with the paper-making processes, beater, press, and the variety of experimental **sheet formations** that were introduced in the papermaking studio. High interest and a strong desire to participate helped the youth engage in planning, focusing, and taking turns as they worked alongside one another. Physical engagement and seeing immediate results anchored their attention. The ability to start over and reuse the pulp at any point minimized the fear of failure and promoted experimentation. Lastly, the hand-as-stencil sheet technique made from T-shirt colors the youth chose and cut together strengthened group belonging while encouraging individual creativity.

Individuals Living with Epilepsy

An on-campus evening workshop series for individuals living with epilepsy was held annually for several years with art therapy faculty and students. The Epi-lepsy Foundation of Wisconsin (http://www.epilepsywisconsin.org) sponsored this series with support from the Lundbeck Studio E project. Epilepsy was often not well understood by the public. For individuals living with epilepsy, "the abrupt and unpredictable occurrence of seizures can ... present many challenges including social barriers" (Havlena & Stafstrom, 2012, p. 65). The series of six to eight weekly workshops introduced different options of art medium, theme, or intention for each session. In the papermaking sessions, participants were in-vited to contribute paper-based items they were ready to let go of or transform, such as a journal entry, news article, or old photo. Materials were then cut up and placed in the pre-pulped 100% cotton rag vat. This space was called the "trans-formation" vat and was available to be shared communally for pulling sheets by all participants. Over the years, several different suggestions for **activating** the handmade paper were offered, such as handmade books, affirmation frames for photos, and using the participants' hands as a stencil for double-couched sheets. During each workshop, the participants selected options relevant to them. The second aim of this series was to increase community awareness and understand-ing of epilepsy. To accomplish this, participants were invited to select artwork from the sessions for a culminating exhibition and reception in the art building's atrium gallery, held in November, which was Epilepsy Awareness Month.

Older Adults

Residents of senior independent and assisted living programs were invited to papermaking workshops as a lifelong learning opportunity. A brief his-tory of papermaking, an overview of the media as a studio art form, and introductory processes generated interest. Older adults have been found to appreciate art processes that build skill, have a product, and can be given to others (Magniant, 2004). Activating handmade papers as a surface for artwork through books, cards, and picture frames also appealed to the activities many older adults valued. Students worked alongside the participants to cut rag, pull sheets, and shape completed art projects. This process fostered intergenerational exchange and understanding.

Transformations with Student and Faculty

In Memory of [My Grandfather]

As a senior, Laura elected to take the papermaking studio art class to deepen the skills she had developed in her previous art therapy courses. For the final paper-making class project, Laura created the piece, *In Memory of [My Grandfather]* (Figure 5.2). Using her grandfather's shirts, she made the paper and covers for two, stacked, bound books. She developed the concept, approached her grand-mother for the shirts, deconstructed them snip by snip, pulped the fabric, and then formed the paper sheets. Fabric pieces of his flannel shirts were incorpo-rated into the book bindings.

Laura's process included many steps, which, when taken together, informed her grief process. She felt her connection to her family strengthen, and her un-derstanding of papermaking as a healing tool grew. The final piece was included in Laura's senior art portfolio. Lastly, Laura created and shared the books with family members.

Abaca Stag

Julianna, a fluent art student who favored three-dimensional media, was intro-duced to papermaking in her art therapy coursework. As part of her independ-ent study project, Julianna produced the sculpture of a stag's head (Figure 5.3). She bent and soldered wire together, stretched wet **abaca** over the form, and

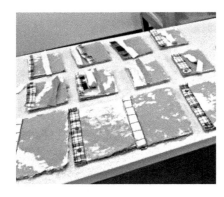

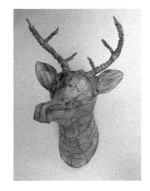

Figure 5.2 Laura's shirt books.   *Figure 5.3 Abaca Stag.*

hung it to dry. Last, she covered it with three layers of linseed oil. This piece ignited Julianna's desire to explore paper as a three-dimensional medium, not just a two-dimensional material. She submitted the sculpture for the annual student art exhibition and included it in her senior art portfolio.

Papermaking in My Garage During the COVID-19 Pandemic

Leah, an art therapy postgraduate, revisited the papermaking process and skills that were part of her undergraduate art therapy coursework. She engaged with papermaking to process and adapt to the isolation of quarantine during the coronavirus (COVID-19) pandemic. Leah chose papermaking over the online world of Internet scrolling, videos, and self-improvement courses. Using plastic tubs as vats, a handmade mould and deckle fashioned from picture frames, and household items, she set up a papermaking station in her garage.

Next, Leah hand tore up old journals containing memories she was ready to process. These journals were reduced to pulp in her blender. To dry the single couched sheets, they were stacked between Pellon® and towels, weighted by books, and placed on her small apartment balcony. Then, Leah hung the sheets on her bulletin board where she could reflect on them as beautiful pieces of abstract art. She also used the sheets to reflect on how the process promoted her growth. Over those months she came to realize though her papermaking how much she had gained from experiences during her post-college years.

Later, Leah carried her pandemic skills into her art classes, offering an outdoor papermaking experience for local home-schooled children. She invited children first to write or draw whatever they wished on pieces of paper to be used for pulp. The children then made paper that would hold a positive message or goal. Leah found the children were willing to try the activity, and they valued the experience whether it was the enjoyment of the process, working together, or sharing their papermaking results.

Papermaking in a Syrian Refugee Camp: Student Research Conference Installation

Emma became invested in expanding their papermaking skills through the studio art course and assisting with workshops. They were accepted for an internship with the Peace Paper Project – a sponsored, social justice and art therapy papermaking workshop with Syrian refugees. The workshop was held at a camp in Germany during the summer of 2017. Emma received internal student research grant assistance from the college to help fund this opportunity. For this project, which received a judge's award at the annual student research conference, Emma created an outdoor simulated refugee camp. Fitted with a tent, cot, personal belongings, and representative composite biographies of refugees, the installation invited viewers to interact with the space and participate in the papermaking processes demonstrated at the site.

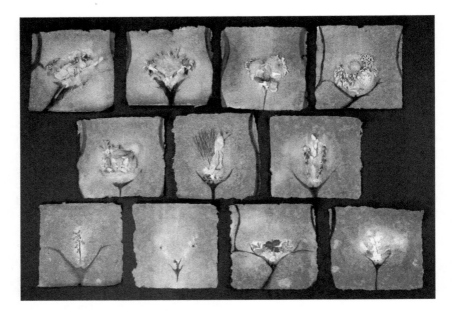

Figure 5.4 Flora Minj.

By the time the camp was held months later in Germany, many refugees and asylum seekers had found assistance and housing. The papermaking processes took place in outdoor spaces provided by local businesses or organizations, as well as indoor locations at artist-affiliated coalitions. As a result of this opportunity, Emma worked with Drew Matott, engaged directly with communities, and studied the therapeutic qualities inherent in papermaking.

Emma's senior portfolio included *Flora Minj* (Figure 5.4) a series created in the papermaking studio class. The series evoked the human form adorned with body hair. It consisted of eleven 7 × 7.5-inch hand-pulled sheets made with a combination of hemp, linen, and newsprint retted in milk. Dried inclusions of dog fur and flowers were added during the cold wall restraint drying process. Each sheet was finished with oil paint and linseed oil.

Papermaking for Legacy and Growth

Brianna, an honors student, was awarded an internal research grant to construct and carry out an eight-week papermaking series that could be sustained by the community partner. This was Brianna's Senior Research project. The grant included funds for basic supplies and materials. The papermaking series worked with older adults living in a long-term care facility. The program investigated how the process of papermaking may help improve the quality of life for people as they aged. Rooted in a sensory-based activity that resulted in work that was wholly handmade, the project provided the residents with direction, motivation, inspiration, and a sense of independence. The project's secondary goal was to adapt the studio art papermaking process, equipment, and fibers for sustainable use in a long-term care facility. Using alternative methods and recipes for paper pulp and ordinary household equipment and tools, residents created unique papers to form cards and books. In a favorite process, inspired by the award-winning children's book, *Miss Rumphius* (Cooney, 1985), residents added wildflower seeds to pulp vats and created cards that loved ones could "plant" in the spring. The process, for many, captured and transformed the aging process into one of legacy and growth.

Papermaking Birds of the Rio Grande Flyway

Inspired by the fall migrations of the sandhill cranes and snow geese, papermaking was used to raise awareness of the Bosque del Apache National Wildlife Refuge (B.d.A.N.W.R.) and the Rio Grande Flyway in New Mexico. Handmade ornaments for the U.S. Fish and Wildlife Service (U.S.F.W.S.) were created statewide as a contribution to the nation's capital holiday decorations (Figure 5.5). Friends of B.d.A.N.W.R. (https://friendsofbosquedelapache.org) sponsored outdoor community papermaking workshops that I led. The role of the Friends

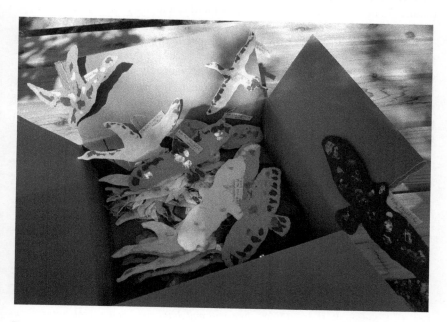

Figure 5.5 Bird ornaments with mica.

supports B.d.A.N.W.R. and promotes appreciation and conservation of wildlife and habitat. For this project, I created stencils of Sandhill cranes, snow geese, hawks, and pintail duck shapes to fit inside moulds and deckles. These stencils represented a few of the more than 450 species of birds of the Rio Grande Flyway. Dehydrated denim and 100% cotton rag obtained from a papermaking supplier made vats of dark blue, light blue, and white pulp. Mica, a naturally occurring mineral of New Mexico, was an optional additive for surface decoration. Mica has iridescent flaking properties that caught the light and adhered well to the wet pulp. These workshops reached across age, gender, and culture to involve a variety of community members and fostered a shared sense of community belonging, accomplishment, and pride.

Conclusion

Although the advantages of a well-equipped, dedicated papermaking studio, especially with a Hollander beater, were evident and inspiring, this was not always available. Everyone profiled in this chapter continued to make paper even when they did not have access to professional studio equipment or a papermaking studio. In addition, they carried the practice into their own art and their work in the community. When a beater was not available, dried **specialty pulp** could be rehydrated and re-mixed. Recycled paper was processed in a blender, upcycled picture frames were modified to serve as moulds and deckles, or affordable student quality tools were used.

Lastly, this chapter has provided a glimpse into the power of papermaking in higher education. This included invigorating an art therapy curriculum, students, their faculty, and the community participants engaged in this papermaking work. As an art therapist and educator, one of the ways I sense my work has made an impact is when the art-making momentum carries on. The essence of papermaking – transformation – once experienced firsthand, ignites imagination and fuels resourcefulness enough to enable more exploration.

References

Ainlay Anand, S. & Gerity, L. (2018). *The legacy of Edith Kramer: A multifaceted view.* Routledge.

Allen, P. B. (1992). Artist in residence: an alternative to "clinification" for art therapists. *Art Therapy, 9*(1), 22–29.

Cooney, B. (1985). *Miss Rumphius.* Puffin Books.

DeLamater, K. (2016, April). Inside Edgewood's paper studio: Handmade paper's role in art therapy. Paperslurry. https://www.paperslurry.com/2016/04/14/inside-edgewood-colleges-paper-studio-handmade-papers-role-in-art-therapy.

Eça, T., & Mason, R. (Eds.). (2008). *International dialogues about visual culture, education, and art.* Intellect Books.

Fenner, L. B. (2016). Constructing the self: Three-dimensional form. In D. E. Gussak & M. L. Rosal (Eds.), *The Wiley handbook of art therapy* (pp. 154–162). Wiley Blackwell.

Gussak, D. E., & Rosal, M. L. (Eds.). (2016). *The Wiley handbook of art therapy*. Wiley Blackwell.

Havlena, J. & Stafstrom, C. (2012). Art therapy with children and adolescents who have epilepsy. In C. Malchiodi (Ed.), *Art therapy and healthcare* (pp. 61–77). The Guilford Press.

Hinz, L. (2016). Media considerations in art therapy: Directions for future research. In D. E. Gussak & M. L. Rosal (Eds.), *The Wiley handbook of art therapy* (pp. 135–142). Wiley Blackwell.

Kramer, E., & Gerity, L. A. (2000). Credo as an artist and as art therapist. In L. A. Gerity (Ed.), *Art as therapy: Collected papers* (pp. 15–19). Jessica Kingsley Publishers.

Magniant, R. C. P. (2004). *Art therapy with older adults: A sourcebook*. Charles C. Thomas.

Malchiodi, C. A. (Ed.). (2011). *Handbook of art therapy* (2nd ed.). Guilford Press.

Moon, C. H. (2001). *Studio art therapy: Cultivating the artist identity in the art therapist*. Jessica Kingsley Publishers.

Moon, C. H. (Ed.). (2010). *Materials & media in art therapy: Critical understandings of diverse artistic vocabularies*. Routledge.

Schwartz, J. B., Rastogi, M., Pate, M. C., & Scarce, J. H. (2021). Undergraduate art therapy programs in the United States survey report. *Art Therapy, 38*(1), 33–41. https://doi.org/10.1080/07421656.2019.1698226.

Timm-Bottos, J., & Reilly, R. C. (2015). Learning in third spaces: Community art studio as storefront university classroom. *American Journal of Community Psychology, 55*, 102–114. https://doi.org/10.1007/s10464-014-9688-5.

6 Voices of the Bereaved

Papermaking for Processing Grief and Loss

Meredith Lin McMackin

This chapter explores the therapeutic aspects of hand papermaking in working with individuals and groups experiencing grief and loss. The author shares her personal experience of loss and engagement with papermaking, along with multiple workshop participants. She briefly examines contemporary themes in grief counseling, including meaning-making and continuing bonds. the author also presents examples of how art therapy addresses those themes. Lastly, through interviews and written questionnaires, individuals describe transforming cloth of significance related to their deceased loved one, and, with those fibers, create a unique commemorative work of art. This chapter also shares how the creative process synthesizes and transforms memories into a symbolic connection that the individuals can keep and cherish.

My Personal Story of Loss

On his second deployment in Iraq, my oldest son and first-born child, was killed, along with another 21-year-old marine, when they rolled over an improvised explosive device (I.E.D.). This shocking and devastating loss left me floundering for some time. The life I had known was gone. I was not the same person. In response, I wanted to do something in my son's honor and to help bring peace to this planet. I searched for several years to find a sense of direction and my role to create healing in this way (Dehart, 2016; McMackin, 2021).

With a lifelong background in the visual arts, I became inspired to pursue art therapy. I loved the idea of using art to help people heal. Then one Spring, I had an opportunity to visit Washington, D.C., and participate in Arts, Military, + Healing: A Collaborative Initiative. This event included a Peace Paper Project workshop. I had heard about this international community arts initiative and how they worked with veterans to make paper from military uniforms. I spent a few hours talking to the facilitators and participants (many of whom were student veterans). I also made my own paper from surplus marine uniforms. I was fascinated by the process, and I felt a special camaraderie with the group. I was hooked!

DOI: 10.4324/9781003216261-9

Upon my return to the university where I was both studying and working, I lobbied the student veterans' center director to bring the Peace Paper Project to campus. I was thrilled when they agreed to sponsor an event. A fellow art therapy student, and a veteran herself, helped rally participation from student veterans. Also, as part of the event, art therapy students on campus learned about papermaking and its therapeutic benefits. The papermaking workshop was a powerful and successful experience for everyone involved. It became an annual event at the university for several years.

During the workshop, I also participated in the papermaking process. I used a piece of my own clothing that held a special connection related to the grief and loss of my son (Figure 6.1). Since I did not have any of my son's uniforms, I pulped the dress I wore to his memorial service. I had not been able to wear it since that day. I put the small pieces of cut clothing into a trough full of water that cycled through a wheel with blades. Then I watched as the fabric was ground and mashed until it became a soft, amorphous pulp suspended in water. The process of cutting, and observing the pulping of the fabric, was an emotional, but fascinating experience. Learning to make my own paper was also fun and forgiving. I felt a sense of release as the fibers were freed from their previous

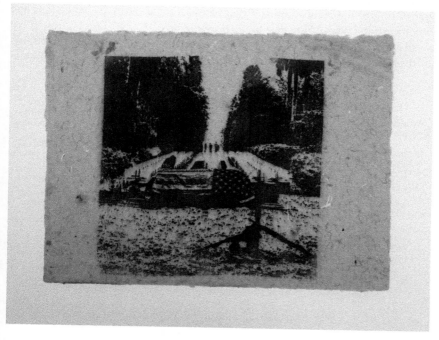

Figure 6.1 Release. Artwork by author.

form and were waiting to be transformed. I also felt a connection to the pulp and the poignant associations it contained.

In addition to my own processing of grief and loss through making paper, I also embarked on doctoral research to further observe student veterans pulp military uniforms in memory of their fellow comrades-in-arms and to redefine themselves as civilians (McMackin, 2016, 2021). Now, several years later as a practicing art therapist and mental health counselor, I have found myself drawn to grief and loss counseling. These paths have brought me back to my original inspiration, to honor my son by helping others, especially those experiencing grief and loss of a loved one.

Processes of Papermaking and Processing Grief and Loss

Figure 6.2 identifies the personal transformation that paralleled with hand papermaking processes in veteran workshops. First, this included advance preparation before attending the workshop. For example, choosing the cloth and personal images to use provided an opportunity to reflect on past relationships and memories. The next step was the cutting and pulping of the cloth. This included deconstructing, recycling, repurposing, cleansing, softening, and additional reflecting. Finally, making the paper art was an experience of creating, transforming, and reconstituting. The process formed creative connections and memories, and bridged the past to the present.

In addition, I recognized that the student veterans were dealing with the loss of their former identities. This included reflecting on friends they had lost in

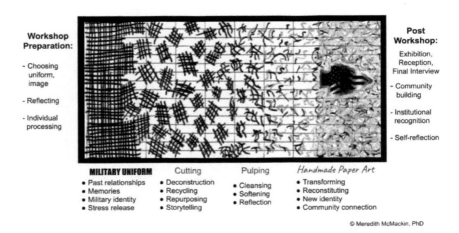

© Meredith McMackin, PhD

Figure 6.2 Paralleling physical papermaking with mental and emotional processing.

war-related deaths. The steps in the papermaking process were applicable to the emotional processes of moving through grief. This involved reflecting and confronting the loss, releasing, and allowing the past to be metamorphosed, yet also retaining and honoring the connection with the deceased. Transforming memorable cloth into paper art provided a tactile, kinesthetic experience to symbolize the individual's emotional transformation.

Reconstructing Meaning through Grief and Loss

As I learned from others about processing grief and loss, I recognized that meaning-making was an integral part of adjusting to loss. In addition, a significant loss often made individuals question their beliefs because the events did not make sense, or they seemed wrong or cruel. Integrating the loss and gaining an understanding of these changes required transformation or reconstruction of one's story. It also required a change in individuals' awareness of life's meaning and value. The act of deconstructing and reconstituting cloth of personal importance provided this transformative process.

A contemporary approach aligned with grief counseling and the transformational process of papermaking is a constructivist perspective. Meaning-making in our lives can be viewed as "constructions of significance" (Neimeyer, 2001, p. 263). The experience of loss becomes woven into the fiber of our lives. Neimeyer suggested that, as in a novel that loses a central character, "the life story disrupted by loss must be reorganized, rewritten, to find a new strand of continuity that bridges the past with the future in an intelligible fashion" (p. 263).

Another example is Viktor Frankl's book, *Man's Search for Meaning* (1959/2006). After surviving multiple concentration camps, Frankl observed and realized that finding meaning in one's life was the most crucial factor in a person's survival. Through all the suffering he experienced and witnessed, Frankl wrote, "In some way, suffering ceases to be suffering at the moment it finds a meaning, such as the meaning of a sacrifice" (p. 113). Even loss can be bearable when there was a felt sense of purpose in one's existence.

Moving through great loss, one has the potential to gain meaningful strength and insight. Research and theory pioneers about post-traumatic growth (P.T.G.), Lawrence Calhoun and Richard Tedeschi have observed through their research that some individuals who have struggled to recover from trauma and loss have also experienced positive changes. They have studied the phenomenon of P.T.G., which resulted in individuals feeling stronger, more resilient, empathic, connected, and a state of resolve in their lives, despite experiencing adversity (Tedeschi et al., 2018). They also concluded that "the transformative nature of loss, then, can be viewed as a process whereby the lives of some people are imbued with an enhanced sense of meaning and purpose" (Calhoun & Tedeschi, 2001, p. 161).

Art Therapy, Meaning-Making, and Processing Grief and Loss

The effectiveness of art therapy for processing grief and loss also showed positive outcomes in relation to meaning-making and creating strong bonds with the deceased (Weiskittle & Gramling, 2018). Art-making supported the concept of adaptive continuing bonds, which include having a symbolic object to represent a loved one's life and, at the same time, aid in accepting their death. Parallel goals between leading theories of grief counseling and art therapy practice both highlight activated change through forming meaningful connections.

For example, Wadeson (2001) described art-making as a way of giving grief form, with the potential for "transfiguration" (p. 59). In this process, something meaningful from the pain of loss can be created. Collaborative art studio environments have often provided a nurturing, creative space for grieving clients to integrate their experience of loss and gain a deeper understanding of themselves (Strouse & LaMorie, 2012). In working with children experiencing loss, Bardot (2008) documented a child's use of art to symbolize feelings in images, translating their loss into meaning and developing resiliency. Additionally, she recognized that the child had "created a foundation of strength from which to draw in the event of future traumas" (p. 184). Rutenberg (2008) engaged patients with a terminal illness and their families in making plaster hand casts as a "way to create a legacy for a terminally ill person and perhaps help patients in preparation for death" (p.110). Casting hands together provided an opportunity to interact and reconnect. After their death, the families had a three-dimensional memento they could touch and hold, as lasting evidence of their loved ones. Junge (1999) also examined the collective contributions of personal losses symbolized in the public memorials of The AIDS Quilt and the Vietnam Memorial Wall. Individual quilt panels sewn together represented lives lost to the AIDS epidemic and mourning objects left at the Vietnam Memorial Wall honored veterans who died in this war. Junge described how the "creativity evoked in the presence of the dead, is the remarkable attempt not only to remember the dead as a process of remembering and marking the meaning of their lives but to create something from that loss" (p. 200).

Shared Stories of Grief and Loss

Years ago, I remember feeling moved when Drew Matott, co-director of the Peace Paper Project, shared his first experience of using papermaking for therapeutic purposes as he spoke to a group before beginning a workshop. He said that making paper from his deceased father's clothing gave him the idea that the process had the potential for healing. Drew shared more about his experience when responding to this author's questionnaire about his loss. His reflections are below.

Drew recalled finding a box of his father's belongings. He looked though some of his father's old clothes and stated, "As soon as my fingers touched the clothes I immediately thought, what if I could turn this into paper?" Drew remembered gathering with his siblings and mother at the dining room table to cut his father's clothes:

My mom shared stories about how she met my father and what it was like being married to a traveling artist, activist, and architect. And my brothers and sister talked about what it was like growing up without a father, always looking to our male instructors in school, coaches, or after-school program coordinators, for a sense of father.

(personal communication)

From that pulped clothing, Drew was inspired to make a book for each member of his family (Figures 6.3 and 6.4). He decided to reprint his father's writings, drawings, photographs, and letters on the handmade paper of each book. Drew discovered:

Through the process of replicating each poem, letter, photo, or drawing, I felt a connection with my father. I felt his presence, I felt that I was making space for him to exist and in this way, I was helping give life to his lost voice.

(personal communication)

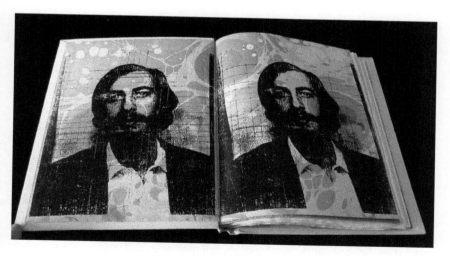

Figure 6.3 Beneath the Bodhi Tree end pages. Artwork by Drew Matott.

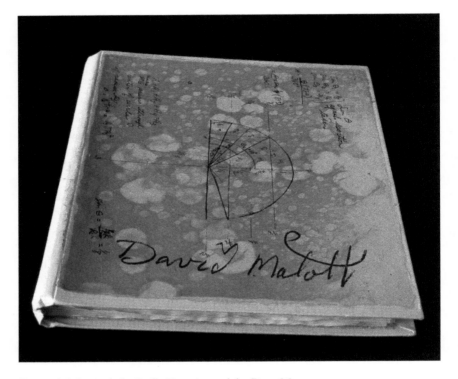

Figure 6.4 Beneath the Bodhi Tree. Artwork by Drew Matott.

Drew's personal papermaking experience also helped inform his future work when facilitating workshops:

> At the core of the workshops, I create a space where individuals are able to create uniquely personal works. I seek to share in the powerful processes that I experienced by creating my father's book and to help **activate** individuals' voices as they work through often painful material.
>
> (personal communication)

With the recent death of my father during the coronavirus pandemic and unable to hold a service, our family came together later to honor the family's patriarch through transforming a couple of his shirts into paper art. I facilitated outdoor papermaking with family members at our home during the summer (Figure 6.5). Similar to what Drew described, while we cut apart and then pulped my father's shirts, we shared special memories and supported each other, acknowledging the loss as well as the love we all felt.

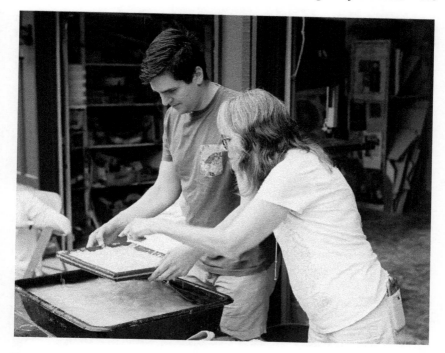

Figure 6.5 Family workshop with author and son. Photograph by Dani Bedard.

To further explore the transformative stories of papermaking with grief and loss, I obtained personal impressions and responses from participants who attended other papermaking workshops I facilitated to memorialize individuals who were dear to them. I designed a questionnaire to gain insight into their papermaking process and to learn about the emotional context of their experiences. The questions asked participants to share a) what was most meaningful about the process, b) what they found surprising, and c) what they thought their deceased family member or close friend might have thought about the process. The voices and individual experiences of participants[1] aligned with studies about the effectiveness of art therapy for processing grief and loss. The responses also supported efforts to find greater meaning in their lives (Weiskittle & Gramling, 2018).

Themes About the Process

Releasing and Deconstruction

When making paper from cloth that held special meaning, typically the first, and often the most difficult step was being willing to let go of the cloth in its original form. Several participants wrote about the difficulty of cutting the garment that related to their past identity, or a loved one that had died. One veteran, Bryan, on his questionnaire wrote about cutting his uniform: "I didn't want to lose any part of it. I was holding onto it emotionally and it was hard destroying it." Juliette, who was grieving the loss of her sister, on her questionnaire wrote about cutting one of her sister's favorite T-shirts:

> The workshop encouraged me to cut up a tee-shirt I held as sacred as well as a bit tainted. It was right for me to make the first cut into it and have the resulting pile be added to the growing piles around the room.
>
> (personal communication)

Juliette added, "I kept one piece intact, it reads 'RELAX.' I still have it. I let the rest of it 'go' during the workshop. I didn't think I ever would" (Figure 6.6). From my own experience, I too, found it hard to cut up my dress associated with my son's death. It was difficult to release it from its existing form, knowing I would not wear it again. Part of me wanted to keep that memory intact, as a tangible object and something I could physically hold on to.

Releasing this symbol provided participants the opportunity to loosen their grip on the past and become open to relating to the memories of their special person in the here and now. The process also allowed the object to be transformed

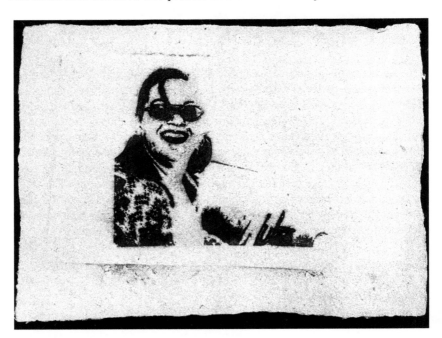

Figure 6.6 Emilie's Smile. Artwork by Juliette.

into something unique, with increased purpose and value. For example, a young widow, Cathy, described the difficulty with the concept of "moving forward." She stated, "to move forward in the way that people mean when they say, 'move on', means things will have to change and that change is devastating." Cathy expressed feeling terrified of this loss. "You don't lose the memories of course, but it takes time, and a lot of tears, to work through this."

As fabric pieces and memories associated with the cloth were placed in the water trough of the **Hollander beater**, they floated free. They were cleansed by the water as they moved around and through the blades of the wheel, grinding, loosening, and releasing the fibers. Eventually, the fabric lost all resemblance to its former state, reduced to a shapeless pulp. Now, the pulp was ready to be transformed into individualized sheets of paper, while still retaining poignant memories. Juliette observed, "the result of feeding fabric strips into the machine was always met with surprise. The subtlety of color, the way it felt in your hands, was beautiful."

Reconstruction and Redefining

Once the pulp was reduced to soft, short, and loose fibers, it was ready to be **pulled** and reconstituted into paper. Lifting the fibers up through the water and onto the surface of the **mould**, the fibers were then transferred and **pressed** onto a surface to dry. This process of transferring the fibers with a rolling movement of the arms and torso, became a rhythmic action. This kinesthetic experience engaged the whole body in the transformative process. After compressing fibers into a sheet of paper, an image could be **pulp printed** onto the paper's wet surface. Some participants used photo silkscreen stencils made from photographs of the person or events they were memorializing. With this method, the selected photograph became part of the paper, intertwined with the treasured fibers. The image gave voice to the paper, visually connecting the person with the cloth to create a cohesive, personal, and expressive work of art. What was once a piece of clothing or other fiber associated with the deceased, was transformed and repurposed, yet it remained connected with the deceased. Bryan, who originally struggled with guilt for cutting his uniform, affirmed, "I am incredibly happy with the end result and do not regret it anymore." In reflection, he wrote about the impact of reconstructing his uniform on his questionnaire:

> The most meaningful part, to me, was the way I got to use my uniform again. Now I have a piece of art hanging on my wall that has meaning. My uniform now has a place of honor on my wall.
>
> (personal communication)

Louise, an artist who was grieving the death of her mother wrote, "The idea of taking a functional garment and turning it into art with the intention of honoring a passed loved one was very meaningful. It unexpectedly opened chambers in the heart. I felt safe to explore those feelings."

Juliette, herself an art therapist, acknowledged on her questionnaire:

I believed fully that the process of making paper from special clothing could help me along my healing journey. The trial and error inherent in the process, the sharing of pulp with others, the selection of images, the sheer power of the Hollander, these aspects and more stood as a metaphor for what I was experiencing inside.

(personal communication)

Sharing Through the Group Experience

In addition to the individual, internal, emotional processing, papermaking in a group setting added multiple positive aspects. Group members supported each other, and conversations often developed through the recollection of memories and experiences. Whether working with a group of veterans, or individuals in a group brought together by loss, they had shared experiences about which to talk. Sometimes those conversations may be lighthearted, pleasant, and include funny moments or memories. One veteran, Bart, wrote how much he enjoyed sharing stories with fellow veterans, including "stories about the person they were honoring, stories about the 'cammies' they were using, and just stories of service in general. It was a great environment to talk about things that you do not get to talk about often."

Juliette described her transformative process and her interactions with others on her questionnaire, saying:

The shirt ceased to be a shirt and became something that a whole roomful of people could ask me if they could "use some of that." In essence, I don't know how many people have paper to this day or how they've used it, that started out as a shirt my sister wore. I feel she's graced many a person this way. She would be so surprised to know that.

(personal communication)

Another veteran, Robert, expressed the most meaningful part of the paper-making process was "partnering and bonding with my fellow veterans. Sharing the stories about the art, why we chose the images we do, and what it meant to us."

Connecting the Deceased to the Experience

In grief theory, recognition of the "potentially healthy role of continued symbolic bonds" (Neimeyer, 2001, p. 3) is valuable when grieving a loved one. To strengthen a sense of continued connection with the deceased through their papermaking experience, I often asked participants what they thought their special person(s) may have felt about the process and the event. In one of my family's workshops, my relative Rick wrote on his questionnaire what he thought his grandfather would think, if he had been there:

> I undoubtedly think he would have been smiling. I think the way in which we honored him, his memory, and ourselves by coming together as a family and doing something simple, yet memorable and profound would have made him proud.
>
> (personal communication)

Other participants expressed feeling a sense of their special person's presence during the creative process. For example, several veterans imagined how their fellow soldiers would feel about their efforts. Bart wrote about his deceased friend, saying, "he would have enjoyed it even more than I did. He was a sentimental guy and artistic. He would have had a great time with it." Bryan thought his friend "would have felt honored." Lastly, Robert on his questionnaire reflected on the loss of many marines in his unit and expressed his appreciation for life:

> What we have is a gift, and I know that if they had it back, they wouldn't waste a second of it. I have tried very hard not to. To enjoy being alive, to be successful, to take care of my mind and body. Because I know they would. This piece of art drives me to do that, so I think they would appreciate that.
>
> (personal communication)

Surprises in the Process

I asked those who had transformed their chosen cloth into paper if anything in the process surprised them. Drew wrote, "Probably the biggest surprise for me was how with each step in the process, I felt a growth, both in my skill set and my emotional well-being." Rick shared, "I was pleasantly surprised that the overall experience brought forth a lot of wonderful memories. Being able to be in the moment of the art process while simultaneously reminiscing was meaningful." The recently widowed Cathy described the process as "a bright spot in a really dark point in my life."

A Reminder of Memories Transformed

For workshop participants, finished artwork became a reminder, not only of the deceased, but also of the transformation and creative process. Contained in the art were materials connected to the memory of the deceased (Figure 6.7).

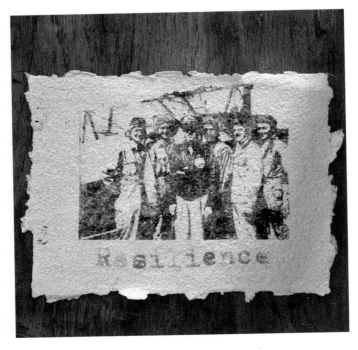

Figure 6.7 The Guardians. Artwork by Rick.

For example, Rick reflected on a specific memory associated with the shirts we pulped belonging to my father on his questionnaire:

> A particular dinner: I couldn't tell you what we ate, but I remember him in his blue shirt reaching for me, as we all joined hands so he could say a quick blessing. A mundane moment for sure, but also an undoubtedly spectacular one that cemented for me during the papermaking process. The fact that I can now look at his upcycled shirt as a piece of art paper, observe the inked image of him from WWII, all while recalling the dinner moment brings me this sort of conflated, layered sense of joy.
>
> (personal communication)

Robert, who said he was initially skeptical of "art therapy" in general, stated on his questionnaire:

> I keep the art in my office now. I look at it every day. It honors people that in some cases, one inch to the left, or 5 minutes earlier, would be here. And maybe I wouldn't. But I am, and that's the world I live in. We have to keep living our lives in a way that honors them and their sacrifice.
>
> (personal communication)

Robert also added that over the years, as he continues to reflect on his experience and his friends that gave their lives, the art has grown in meaning (Figure 6.8).

Drew shared how his book made from his father's clothing became a force for healing relationships years after his father's death. He described how the book helped his uncle heal his strained relationship with his brother (Drew's father). He reflected on his uncle's emotional reaction to the book and how it inspired him to share stories of growing up as brothers, as well as his regrets and emotions about his brother's death, and their lack of reconciliation. Drew wrote on his questionnaire:

> I felt that my uncle was able to use the book, and in some part our meetings as a way to remember my father, bring him back, fill that dark hole with positive memories and smooth out his sense of regret, loss, and remorse.

(personal communication)

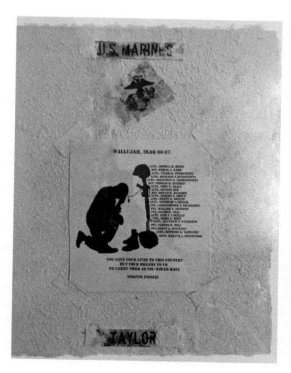

Figure 6.8 Artwork by Robert.

Conclusion

In reflecting on this chapter, I was moved by the willingness of participants to share personal feelings and experiences related to grief and loss, the papermaking process, and art. The descriptions revealed processing grief in physical and visible forms. Through making paper with clothing of personal importance, these individuals were able to transform their memories into a lasting symbolic work of art.

Although each participant had different relationships with the deceased, there were common emotional responses within the group experience as well as internal meaning-making with the papermaking process. Individuals described creating meaning from remnants of past associations. Through this process, they strengthened their connection with the deceased. Synthesizing and reconstructing meaningful memories, the art became the symbol of that metamorphosis. Fibers bonded to form a surface embedded with memories and meaning. And this became a work of art. As Louise, the daughter grieving the loss of her mother recognized, "I am an artist and believe in transformation of emotion and spirit into tangible form."

Note

1 Participant names associated with the questionnaire responses were all changed to pseudonyms to provide privacy.

References

Bardot, H. (2008). Expressing the inexpressible: The resilient healing of client and art therapist. *Art Therapy, 25(*4), 183–186. http://www.doi.10.1080/07421656.2008. 10129547.

Calhoun, L. G., & Tedeschi, R. G. (2001). Posttraumatic growth: The positive lessons of loss. In R. A. Neimeyer (Ed.), *Meaning reconstruction and the experience of loss* (pp.157–172). American Psychological Association. https://doi.org/10.1037/10397-008.

Dehart, J. (2016, March). The Peace Paper Project weaves veterans into the community fabric. *Tallahassee Magazine.* https://www.tallahasseemagazine.com/the-peace-paper-project-weaves-veterans-into-the-community-fabric.

Frankl, V. E. (2006). *Man's search for meaning.* Beacon Press. (Original work published 1959)

Junge, M. B. (1999). Mourning, memory, and life itself: The AIDS Quilt and the Vietnam Veterans' Memorial Wall. *The Arts in Psychotherapy, 26*(3), 195–203. https://doi.org/ 10.1016/S0197-4556(99)00007-6.

McMackin, M. L. (2016). *Assessing the value of creative arts workshops and hand papermaking for student veterans in transition.* ProQuest Number: 10161214.

McMackin, M. (2021). Hand papermaking with student veterans. In R. Mims (Ed.), *Art therapy with veterans* (pp. 57–77). Jessica Kingsley Publishers.

Neimeyer, R. A. (2001). The language of loss: Grief therapy as a process of meaning reconstruction. In R. A. Neimeyer (Ed.), *Meaning reconstruction and the experience of loss* (pp. 261–292). American Psychological Association.

Rutenberg, M. (2008). Casting the spirit: A handmade legacy. *Art Therapy, 25(3)*, 108–114. http://www.doi.org/10.1080/07421656.2008.10129592.

Strouse, S., & LaMorie, J. H. (2012). The art studio process. In R. A. Neimeyer (Ed.), *Techniques of grief therapy: Creative practice for counseling the bereaved* (pp. 226–228). Routledge.

Tedeschi, R., Shakespeare-Finch, J., Taku, K., & Calhoun, L. (2018). *Posttraumatic growth: Theory, research, and applications*. Routledge.

Wadeson, H. (2001). Art, death, and transfiguration. *Art Therapy, 18*(1), 56–60. https://doi.org/10.1080/07421656.2001.10129448.

Weiskittle, R. E., & Gramling, S. E. (2018). The therapeutic effectiveness of using visual art modalities with the bereaved: A systematic review. *Psychology Research and Behavior Management, 11*, 9–24. https://doi.org/10.2147/PRBM.S131993.

Part III

Papermaking as Personal Voice

7 Papermaker Reflections
Stories of Change, Growth, and Creativity

Courtney Bowles and Mark Strandquist, Jennifer L. Davis, Tom Lascell, Nathan Lewis, Annie McFarland, Rachel Mims, Erin Mooney-Simkus, Yaslin M. Torres-Peña, Denise R. Wolf, Eli Wright

This chapter offers a collection of ten first-person essays. Each gives a voice to how papermaking has empowered a personal story of change, growth, transformation, and creative expression. Voice can be defined as a vehicle providing communication of internal and external viewpoints, feelings, thoughts, and encounters. Voice can emerge in the form of spoken and unspoken language through the following words, conversations, advocacy, writing, storytelling, poetry, music, and art. To be heard and seen as a papermaker can create a source of raw empowerment connection, and validation for the individual. This experience is valuable to finding and restoring one's sense of self by exploring aspirations and acknowledging human experiences of challenge and triumph.

Papermaking's meaningful associations with what has been chosen for **pulping** is another means to find one's voice by acting and imagining new possibilities. With papermaking's distinct transformative methods, an opportunity exists to engage with and share personal, communal, and socially informed narratives, implications, and experiences beyond words. The expressions and images that form this chapter assert unique papermaking narratives as students, studio artists, educators, therapists, activists, veterans, art facilitators, and community organizers.

*

The People's Paper Co-op
Courtney Bowles and Mark Strandquist

"These records hold us back, they hold us down. Like a tail, they keep tripping us up; as we try to move our lives forward, they come back to haunt us."
— *Anonymous clinic participant, age 28*

First, you hear music.
Soulful sounds burst through the door. *Wait, is this a legal clinic?*
You're here because you're hoping to get your criminal record cleared, and as you step off the street and into North Philadelphia's Village of Arts

DOI: 10.4324/9781003216261-11

and Humanities (https://villagearts.org), you're welcomed by one of the formerly incarcerated leaders at the People's Paper Co-op (P.P.C.) (http://peoplespaperco-op.com). The P.P.C. fellows that greet you will help you get seated, get settled, get your paperwork started, and make sure you know, that they know, that this is tough but can also be liberating. Credible peer messengers can completely shift someone's experience. There will be other sounds in the room too, including people laughing, crying, smiling, while tearing up documents, and the familiar whirl of a blender. Smoothies? Milkshakes? Sort of, you'll find out about that later. Sitting with upwards of a hundred other community members with criminal records you look around and see walls full of supportive art created by P.P.C. fellows. Posters with portraits and text, with statements like: "Stop Arresting Us, You Should Invest in Us," "We Are Not Our Mistakes!," "Don't Let Your Past Hold You Back," "Be the Mentor You Wish You'd Had," and "Together, We'll Make This World Better."

Oh, and there's free food, lots of it, all made by neighborhood hero, culinary wizard, and Village Elder in Residence, Ms. Nandi.

To sum it up, it's not your typical social service space. As one community participant said about their experience, "I came not knowing a single person and I'm leaving feeling like I just went to a family reunion."

More than 70 million people in the U.S. have a criminal record. This is close to 1 in 3 adults and more than the entire population of France. These records disproportionately impact communities of color and create obstacles to employment, housing, education, social mobility, and other basic human rights, while shackling people to their past (The Sentencing Project, 2015). In Pennsylvania, any charges, regardless of conviction, stay on a person's record (Pennsylvania General Assembly, 2022). In North Philly, The Village sits at the intersection of three police districts. The neighborhood has suffered from over-policing and long-term disinvestment, and the arrest rate in this area is higher than in much of the city (Philadelphia Police Department, 2022). Many individuals in the 19133 zip code are impacted by the lasting ramifications of criminal records (themselves, their friends, and loved ones) and access to free expungement (clearing or cleaning up criminal records) in the neighborhood is very much needed. With Lead P.P.C. fellow Faith Bartley, we have directed the People's Paper Co-op, which connects formerly incarcerated individuals with lawyers, artists, and activists, to co-design these legal clinics. This project has turned often dehumanizing social service spaces into peer-led environments full of real and symbolic transformation, where papermaking has been a huge part.

Going through one's criminal record can be a traumatizing experience – revisiting some of the darkest days of an individual's life. In response, we wanted to design and offer a cathartic and healing ritual for participants. Papermaking was the perfect transformative medium. After lawyers work with each clinic participant to begin the expungement process, interested participants work with P.P.C. fellows to tear up their criminal records and put them in blenders (those paper smoothies you heard about earlier) to create new sheets of handmade paper (Figure 7.1). With their criminal records **pulped**, participants then write statements in response to the prompt, "Without my criminal record, I am ..." and take a Polaroid portrait (a "reverse mugshot"), both of which they embed into the new sheet of paper they have made. These new sheets of paper are physical representations of transformed records and act as a blank slate for people to rewrite their future narratives.

We designed a papermaking system that was both portable (one that could be set up in church basements, sidewalks, and community centers) and as accessible as possible. We learned papermaking from online videos, bought thrift-store blenders, collected a lot of brightly colored aprons, and built our frames from scrap wood. To ensure the process was very hands-on during the portable workshops, each step was taught (oftentimes by someone who had just learned) from pulping to **pressing** the sheets by hand, creating a **post** with **couched** sheets, and hanging up used **Pellon®** to dry. It was important that the papermaking was a one-to-one experience, and that people knew they could use materials they might already have around their houses – that almost anything can be transformed into something new, beautiful, and meaningful.

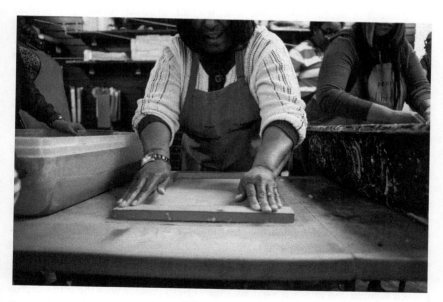

Figure 7.1 Papermaking at an expungement intake. Photo by Mark Strandquist and courtesy of the People's Paper Co-op.

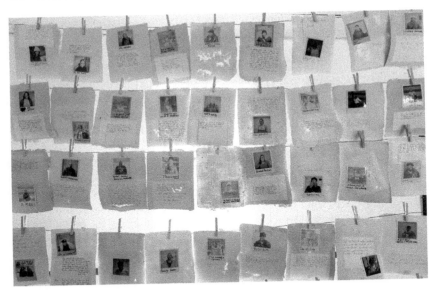

Figure 7.2 Criminal record quilt pieces. Photo by Mark Strandquist and courtesy of the People's Paper Co-op.

Hundreds of people have made what we call "criminal record quilt pieces" (Figure 7.2). The growing collection has been displayed in subsequent legal clinics and exhibited in the Philadelphia Museum of Art, Philadelphia's City Hall, churches, universities, galleries, and more. These exhibits have served as empowering reflections for community members affected by the criminal justice system while reaching tens of thousands of viewers in public-facing displays, press releases, and events connected with the artwork. We wanted the work to have real impacts on those we were collaborating with, as well as helping to transform society's narratives around the criminal legal system.

Partnerships power all our work. The expungement clinics have been made possible only through collaboration with legal advocates at Philadelphia Lawyers for Social Equity (http://www.plsephilly.org), Community Legal Services (http://clsphila.org), and the support of countless volunteers and law students. As the program has continued to adapt and evolve, the transformative process of papermaking has remained an integral part of our work. P.P.C. continues to use papermaking as a tool for participants to process personal trauma while creating powerful art that can reach both broad and specific audiences.

Each spring since 2018, the P.P.C. has worked with a cohort of justice-involved women and artists from across the U.S. to partner with the Philadelphia Community Bail Fund (http://www.phillybailout.org) on their Black Mama's

Bail Out. Each year the initiative raises money to bail out Black moms and caregivers, bringing them home to be with their loved ones and communities in time for Mother's Day. The P.P.C. fellows and collaborating artists create posters, prints, shirts, and public art that amplify the urgent messages the women wanted to convey, help the bail fund visualize their campaign, raise funds, and advocate the end of cash bail. The media and messaging that power the poster campaign were made by women in re-entry themselves, who know the issues better than anyone. The resulting images were screen printed on handmade paper the women made from their criminal records and the prints were sold as a fundraiser for the bail fund. In just three years, the artwork raised over $175,000 for local and national bail funds. For centuries, artists have made art about the idea of freedom; the women in the P.P.C. have used their art literally to free people.

Papermaking has and continues to be an incredibly powerful medium for us and our collaborators. Full of agency, magic, and transformative poetry, the project showcases new models of collective art-making. The impact ripples out in concentric circles, from an intimate and cathartic vehicle for healing and self-representation to art pieces, exhibits, and campaigns that transform more than pulp and water.

*

A Personal Journey through Cancer, Papermaking, and Self-Transformation

Jennifer L. Davis

Good stories have a beginning, a middle, and an end. This is a story of brokenness, resilience, courage and strength, and transformation. My story begins with breaking down. Before the transformation from **rag** to paper can start, the process of making paper also requires that the fibers be broken down by the bladed roll of the **Hollander beater**. Before my transformation, I, too, had been broken down.

I found the lump on the left side of my left breast. I wasn't too concerned because I had had my mammogram less than a year earlier. My annual woman's exam was in a few weeks, and I would be sure to mention it. My doctor was somewhat concerned and suggested I have another mammogram. A few days after the mammogram I had an ultrasound and biopsy. I said to my doctor, "You see this a lot. Do you think this is cancer?" His opinion was that it was.

In the middle of teaching fourth-grade reading, I received a phone call that confirmed what I had suspected. I had cancer. I drove to where my mother was working and would be waiting for the results. We hugged and cried. That afternoon I did one of the hardest things I have ever done. I told my 13-year-old daughter and my 10-year-old son that I had breast cancer. I looked around the room at my children, my mother, and my two closest friends and told them how much I loved them and that I was going to be okay. Then my children and I packed up our car and went to a weekend bike race in which I and many other cyclists peddled and carried our mud-ridden mountain bikes through the deepest, stickiest, muddiest Kansas singletrack I'd ever encountered. I knew that if I could grind my way to the finish line, then I could beat cancer.

The days and weeks that followed were a whirlwind of meetings and emotions. The first surgery for treatment and my life was a bilateral mastectomy with reconstruction. This eight-hour surgery removed all my breast tissue along with the cancerous tumors and replaced that space with carbon fiber expanders that prepared my skin for implants later. This procedure occurred ten days before my 40th birthday. I had never experienced such pain as I did from the mastectomy. I required assistance in showering and washing and combing my long hair. I had four drains attached to tubes that were inserted through holes in my chest. I attached and hid these drains in my clothing and wore specially made tank tops just for this purpose.

The days of waiting for the pathology report were agonizing. I was confident I could beat stage one or even stage two cancer. I would not allow myself to even consider anything worse. Finally, the pathology report was in. I had estrogen and progesterone receptor-positive invasive ductal carcinoma stage three. They found not one, but two tumors and the cancer had begun to spread. The next step was chemotherapy. The poison that would kill my cancer would be administered through a port surgically implanted into my chest wall and directly connected to my jugular vein. My prescribed chemotherapies were meant to kill any cancer left in my body that the mastectomy could not remove. The day after each chemo I would return for a Neulasta shot, a drug that increased the production of white blood cells. For me, this was a painful process. To prevent nausea, I was given more drugs. All my hair fell out. My face became swollen, my skin was severely dry, and my fingernails and toenails stopped growing. My mouth was sensitive, and food tasted like chemicals. I was put into instant menopause, which created many more undesirable effects. Midway through my treatments, I was in a car accident. My injuries were painful but superficial. This was one more blade on the beater, trying to break me down.

After six rounds, one every three weeks, chemotherapy was complete. I had a surgical procedure that removed the expanders and put saline implants in their place. Then the preparation for 30 days of radiation began. I was crudely tattooed and fitted with a special form that kept my body in place to ensure precise radiation. My skin became severely burned. The radiation caused a painful condition called a capsular contracture in which the scar tissue surrounding the implants hardened. I had yet further surgery that removed the implants. The last surgery I had was a hysterectomy. The type of cancer I had was fed by estrogen and progesterone and this procedure helped reduce the risk of a recurrence. I was also at high risk for ovarian and uterine cancers. This surgery eliminated that chance. To me, my body looked and felt like it had been through the beater. I was tired of being cut up. I wanted to feel whole.

It was not long after I had finished all my treatments that I was introduced to the papermaking process. With the assistance of Drew Matott and the Peace Paper Project, I began breaking down my chosen fibers. I cut up my now worthless bras and the drain tanks that had held the post-operative drains. Cutting the fibers to prepare them for the beater was tedious and strenuous. It was a slow process. The straps, clasps, and wires had to be cut out. The remaining fabric was cut with scissors into small postage stamp size pieces. Over the years, I have tried to find easier, more efficient ways of cutting up the fiber. There just does not seem to be any way around it. Sometimes, you must do hard things. These small pieces were placed into the Hollander beater. I also saved a few lacy bits from my bras and mixed them into the pulp.

The sound of the machine macerating the fiber was loud. As the fibers began to break and the roller was lowered toward the bedplate, it was even louder. At times, I became attuned to the sound, and only when the roller was raised towards the end of the process did I realize how loud it was. I appreciated the quiet calm peace that followed.

The **pulp** was not what I expected. The black, white, and pink fibers mixed to create a soft pink with small flecks of the original colors and lacy pieces. Again and again, I repeatedly strained the pulp from the **vat** with the **mould** and **deckle** and couched the pulp into 9 × 12-inch pieces. My stack of about 50 sheets was then **pressed** and **dried**.

I loved this part of papermaking, especially on a hot Kansas day. Water soaked through my clothes as I transferred the sheet to the stack. When the stack started to curve, and the pulp sheet began to break I knew it was time to move it to the press. The stack was sandwiched between boards and rivulets of water flowed as the press was lowered. It was now paper. The wet sheets were laid to dry, which in July would only take a few hours. Once the paper was dried it was peeled off the **interfacing**. This was the first time the qualities of the finished paper could be examined. No two pieces were ever the same. There were variations in colors and textures. Water, fibers, and my hand movements created subtle nuances in each sheet. Worn-out beaten rag created paper that was beautiful and looked new again. It was transformed.

I found gratitude in taking something worn, tired, hurt, damaged, hopeless, worthless, and making it new and beautiful: making it whole again. Papermaking and creating were healing for me. Through the process, I found a sense of calm and presence in the moment. This presence sometimes brought painful awareness. An awareness that built strength and resilience. Resilience built hope that heals. I started to recognize this change in myself.

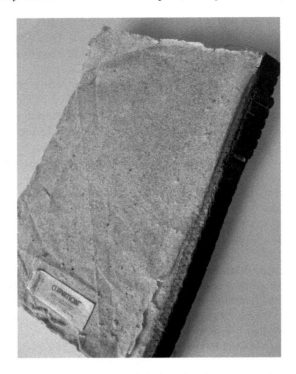

Figure 7.3 Book made from my bras and drain tanks. Bra straps and tags were used in the binding.

When the paper that I made that day was finished, it was strong, beautiful, and full of potential. The sheets were bound into a book (Figure 7.3) which contained photos and stories of my journey through cancer (Figure 7.4). This story, *my* story, however, was not complete. Like the paper, I was being transformed. Like the paper, I was not meant to have a single purpose. I started to feel beautiful again and to reimagine my life.

I became passionate about the papermaking process. I learned as much as I could about it and I acquired my own Hollander beater. I gave classes and workshops. I taught other cancer survivors how to make their own paper. I led a papermaking workshop for an addiction recovery center. I taught others how to bind books from their papers. I made paper with my students. I created books, collages, and a mural from handmade paper. I started to show my work in small regional venues and art markets (Figure 7.5). I began selling my artwork. Some of the money I made helped pay toward my astronomical medical debt. I also made a switch from teaching fourth grade to an elementary art classroom.

My story doesn't have a beginning, a middle, and an end. My story has a beginning, a middle, and a *new beginning*. After 26 years of teaching, I quit my

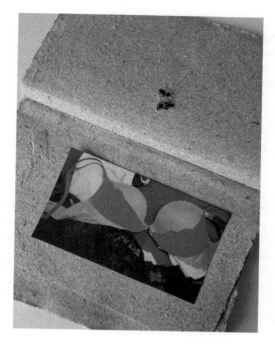

Figure 7.4 My bras before they were cut up to produce the book's paper.

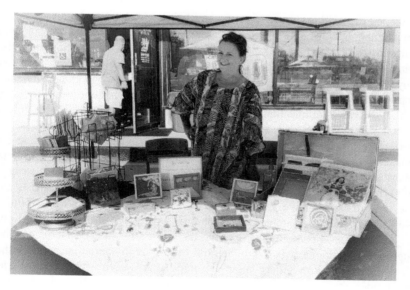

Figure 7.5 Showing my artwork at an art market in Derby, Kansas.

job and sold my house. I changed my career path to pursue a second Master's degree in Marriage and Family Therapy. I will hold space for others as they process their pain and trauma. I will help them find courage, strength, and resilience for their own transformative new beginning by incorporating the cathartic act of papermaking and art into my practice.

*

From Photographer to Papermaker and Book Artist: A Creative Odyssey

Tom Lascell

I am a papermaker and book artist. But that's not where I started. I began my creative journey by looking through the lens of a camera, capturing snippets of time, often in a romantic style. I was more interested in my own aesthetic interpretation of a scene than an impartial rendering of time and space. To me, an effective photograph emitted that emotional "pinprick". It crystallized a changed and somewhat charged reality. It had a life of its own. If I was successful, I conveyed to others what I first saw before I raised the camera to my eye. This was that magical moment that first drew me to photography. I found it in my viewfinder; I found it in the developing tray.

Photography and the Creative Process

I learned the craft, as many have, by emulating Ansel Adams' majestic nature images and, later, by exploring Aaron Siskind's abstract images of peeling paint. But mostly I learned by making lots of mistakes: thousands of images that became more technically precise over time but fell short of greatness. Occasionally, I stumbled upon something special. What made that one image shine and separate itself from the mediocre and mundane? What made it worth framing? Ah … the essential question. Having once found success I tried to repeat it. If I remained there too long, my creativity became stuck; I became engrossed in perfecting my craft. Thankfully, I have been able to realize, "I've made that image before." I could continue to do the same thing, again and again, or metaphorically give myself a kick by exploring something new. That eternal struggle of perfecting our craft vs. vision is, I think, a common challenge for artists. For me, they go hand in hand. Learning new skills opened new creative possibilities. New ideas demanded I improve my technical skills to better express what I saw.

So how does a photographer get into the paper arts? In my experience, photographers traditionally had two methods to display or share their work: either as framed prints in a gallery show or compiled as a coffee table book. I tried to broaden my perspective. I had been exposed to alternative photographic processes. I relished the handcrafted feel of contact printing my images under the noontime sun. What seemed a natural progression to me was to create my own paper on which to print my images. Instead of confining myself to traditional commercial papers, I made my own. My biggest challenge was to create a smooth surface on which to paint the light-sensitive **emulsion** so I could fully render the details found in my negatives.

Finding Inspiration in an Artist Collective

At the time, I was working out of the Green Door Studio (http://www.peace-paperproject.org/greendoorstudio), an artist collective, in Burlington, Vermont, (Figure 7.6). I shared a darkroom with three others; the rest of the studio was comprised of painters, musicians, and papermakers of a younger generation. I decided to join the collective to be around creative people. I didn't want to get into an artistic rut by working from my home studio. I preferred to invest in other creatives, hopefully gaining from an idea thrown out in an entirely different context. I organized my negatives for printing at home, then traveled three hours to print my images in the darkroom during a marathon session. I worked late into the night until my chemistry was exhausted, then joined others in the studio as music

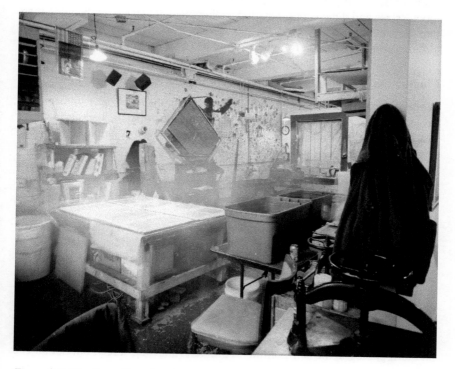

Figure 7.6 The Green Door Studio.

blared, paper pulp was beaten, and sheets were **pulled**. Creative ideas flowed. I started hanging out with papermakers, learned the craft, and experimented with other papers suitable for printing and moulding, **broadsides,** and book covers.

Papermaking and the Creative Process

I started with straight linen paper, but it was too porous and prone to wrinkling. I then experimented with cotton rag, but it didn't hold up well to the lengthy water bath needed to wash photographic prints. I've had good success with the cotton/**abaca** mix with a light external **slurry** after the sheets have dried. My latest formula comprises white cotton rag and abaca in a 9:1 ratio.

I found that printing on handmade papers added an extra subtlety and depth to my image-making. The texture can feel like canvas, the deckle edges provide a visual frame. Once I dipped my hands into the paper pulp, I was hooked. The same tactile pleasure I found in the darkroom transferred to pulling sheets of paper from the vat.

I also experimented with wrap-around book covers. They needed to be thicker, stronger, and more intriguing than a traditional sheet of paper. I added natural fibers to my mix, often layering them on my pulled sheet. I worked in unique sizes and dimensions. I started adding plant ephemera, embedding them into the wet pulp. When dried, the plants were held tight. My initial foray into pulling paper sheets as a printing substrate had found a third dimension.

Finding Deeper Meaning in Papermaking

While working with veterans from Afghanistan and Iraq at the Combat Paper Project (http://www.combatpaper.org), it became clear that the message was not just in the image printed on a sheet of handmade paper. The paper itself had a story to tell, perhaps even more compelling than the printed image or text. The story in the fiber became the underlying mantra (Valentino, 2013). For the veterans working at the Green Door Studio, this was manifested as making paper out of their military uniforms to tell their personal stories, as a means of personal transformation and to unlock their memories and express their feelings of trauma or camaraderie. But that wasn't my story. As a Vietnam-era veteran from a different generation, I was in a different place. I'd been drafted out of college after serving in the Peace Corps. I hated how the army stripped me of my individuality, from the very first day, in their attempt to turn me into a soldier.

I experimented with making paper pulp casts of my face from a plaster mould, using different colored pulps, and embedding ephemera from my service in the army (Figure 7.7). What better way to tell my personal story, to reclaim my identity than my face rendered in paper inserted with memories, artifacts, and torn photographic self-portraits? An interesting step surely, but not an end in itself. But the mantra was still cogent. How could I incorporate the fiber as a fundamental part of the story I wanted to tell?

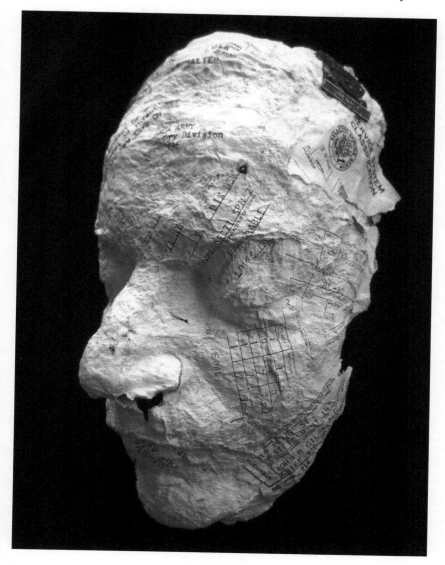

Figure 7.7 Paper mask with embedded military ephemera.

Using Raw Fibers for Personal Art-making

My papermaking skills were grounded in the traditional **Western-style**, but I've also experimented with making paper in the **Eastern-style**, which uses a bamboo mat as the mould, washing the long **bast fibers** back and forth into large, ultra-thin sheets. I learned to **cook** natural fibers and to slow the drainage of the pulp.

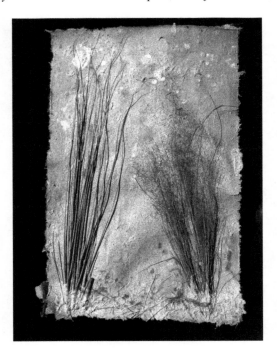

Figure 7.8 Carolina.

By using my technique of placing natural plant ephemera into the pulled sheet, I created large natural pastoral pieces; I celebrated nature by using plants from each of the four seasons. I also created an edition depicting the marsh of coastal South Carolina. The base sheet was made from spartina grass and pulled in the Eastern-style on a sugetta. The ever-present "pluff mud" of the marsh's floor was represented by native sweetgrass (Figure 7.8). Each of those pieces was given to environmentalist friends who devoted their lives to conserving the marsh.

Another time, after attending the wedding of my cousin, I harvested flowers from the bridal bouquet and reception table centerpieces to create a memento for the bride and groom (Figure 7.9). I recreated the bridal bouquet crafted from rose petals and eucalyptus with embedded rose blossoms. The wedding invitation was embedded in the back. I also made an accompanying piece celebrating the groom's mother; she had died earlier in the year and thus was absent from the wedding. There was an arrangement of her favorite flowers on a grand piano at the reception in her memory. The basic sheet of paper I made was from ferns and wildflowers, pulled over sheet music of her favorite hymn, and embedded with a selection of wildflowers. Incorporated into the back was a memorial from the wedding announcement. She was a piano teacher and church organist by profession. The story was in the fiber.

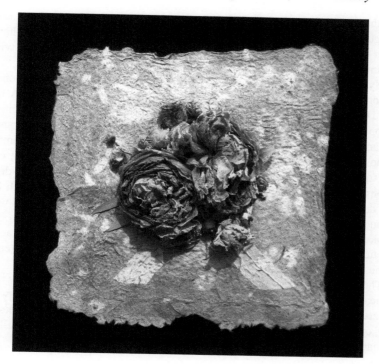

Figure 7.9 Mother's Wedding Flowers.

Merging Papermaking and Photography through Book Art

Creativity doesn't always appear in an orderly fashion, with one project leading directly to another. While I continued to shoot pictures, I also began making **artist books** to give a greater voice to my photographic images. As I became more confident with my skills as a papermaker, I began incorporating elements of hand papermaking into my book art.

My first book was a study of faces, a hard-bound coffee table book of black and white images taken in the Katmandu bazaar. The only text was on the fly-leaf, just enough to set the stage. I have learned that every choice matters: each element must work in harmony and support each other. I usually start with the content. From there I can make considered decisions about size and shape, paper and typeface, binding and layout, illustrations, and white space. My second, *Rustic Weather*, made in collaboration with Drew Matott, featured my black and white images of weathered wood arrayed in an accordion fashion. The **letter-pressed** text was minimal, just enough to encourage page turns. As the viewer, you could choose which images to show in a series, then re-fold the accordion in a different manner, and you were rewarded with a completely new visual array.

Another book, *Conversation with Grey Wolf* featured a dialogue between seeker and guide. My black and white images illustrated the back-and-forth exchange, water images for the guide, and forest images for the seeker. I bound it with a handmade wrap-around cover made from cotton, abaca, and blue iris.

My latest project was inspired by the *Thanksgiving Address* of the Mohawk Nation (Stokes, 1993). I imagined what it might have looked like in book form at the time of first contact with European explorers. It is an invocation recited at the opening of any significant gathering. It gave thanks to the spirits and ancestors and served to unite the people by inviting participants to focus on a common purpose. The handcrafted pages were made from "three sisters" (beans, corn, and squash) paper for the text. Translucent cattail paper displayed hand-drawn glyphs. End pages were made from sweetgrass. My book featured birch bark and deerskin covers, all held together with a simple stab binding. The wrap-around dust cover was made from black wool fabric, reminiscent of a trade blanket. Page markers were crafted from deerskin thongs, adorned with acorns and turkey feathers. I chose to render their spirit in book form, paying attention to the technology and materials available circa 1600.

Throughout my personal journey, I have come to realize that creativity is not a linear progression. There is no one path to follow. We all start from right where we are. The next step may depend on an external spark, a change of perspective, or simply imagining something anew. Maybe it's just a question of asking, "What if…?"

*

Beating the War: Fighting Militarism through Papermaking

Nathan Lewis

Occasionally I'm asked: "How did you get into papermaking?" I usually take a breath and run a few calculations in my head concerning time, mood, and the inquisitor's level of genuine interest. If I was short on time or didn't feel like going deep into politics or my life story, the short answer was usually "a friend taught me." Typically, the longer answer was, "I got into papermaking through the U.S. army." From there the conversation either wandered into the technical weeds of a 2,000-year-old craft (Hunter, 1974), or it veered into the politics of the War on Terror (Richissin, 2004).

Of course, you cannot join the U.S. army to be a papermaker. Last I heard they were starting to incorporate yoga into boot camp, and I have met at least one active-duty U.S. army artist whose job was to sketch and paint daily life in the military and in war zones (U.S. Army Center of Military History, 2021). I didn't receive training or encouragement to become an artist in the military. The home I grew up in valued the two forms of art I think were the most available and appreciated by the working class: music and movies. Nobody in my family called movies "films." Nobody in my family went to art galleries, talked about art, or called themselves an artist. Going to school to be an artist was considered a riskier and more dubious life decision than joining the military. Growing up in a poor rural community, I was more likely to be sitting behind the canvas door of a Humvee with an M-16 rifle than in front of a stretched canvas with a paintbrush.

The story of how and why I joined the military I think was a typical one of many young Americans. Personal goals intersected with vague patriotism. Towards the end of high school, I was in the guidance counselor's office. Replying to an open-ended question on a form, I wrote I would like to go to college and work with computers. Since I misspelled both college and computer, the guidance counselor slid an army brochure across the desk. "There's jobs with computers in the army, and they give you money for college," they said. I was primed for later in the year when the recruiters called.

The terrorist attacks of September 11, 2001, happened during my first week of basic training. I was fresh out of high school and learning simple army private skills like marching, saluting, and boot shining. My days were tough, chaotic, and painful. On that day, the hundred or so recruits I was with were herded into a large room after our evening meal. A decrepit projection TV was wheeled out and we watched the towers fall on CNN several dozen times. As if out of a movie, a large and intense drill instructor stood before us and told us we better pay attention and learn well. He guaranteed we would all be going to war. We should consider ourselves lucky, as he hadn't yet had the pleasure. Six months later I was in an artillery unit deploying to invade Iraq. I had my doubts about the wisdom or morality of the Iraq War, but in the end, I went along with it and did my tour. About halfway through, I decided I was done. When I got home, I let my enlistment contract expire and left the military.

In the military, I collected a steel shipping container full of stories, intense experiences, reflections, regrets, accomplishments, and travels. I participated, willing or unwillingly, in significant historical events, international piracy, personal growth, and debasement. I became strange and estranged, which was to say, I would never again be a civilian. Any veteran courageous and strong enough to open this shipping container and create art with the shit and gold found inside had plenty of meaning and inspiration to fuel a lifetime of creative endeavors.

As I took classes at a community college and worked jobs, I watched the war I just returned from turn into a horrible mess. I'd sit in the cafeteria eating lunch and the televisions had me transfixed. I'd watch Fallujah burn between Psych 101 and Spanish class. After Anthropology I would stop for a quick update on Abu Ghraib. After finishing my homework I'd stop for a late-night snack and a few minutes of a truck convoy being burned. There was no moment of epiphany or singular thing that turned me against the war. There was also no defiant moment where I became an activist and spoke out or did anything against the war. Slowly I went from complaints and grievances to action and determination.

At first, the only anti-war movement I found was made up of large national protest marches. One time, my desert camouflage caught the attention of some Vietnam veterans. A rough-looking dude in head-to-toe olive drab fatigues, festooned in colorful buttons bearing peace signs and slogans, came up and hugged me. He said, "Welcome Home, Brother" and that was it. It felt like I had just been initiated into a different world where veterans spoke, thought, and acted differently. These were the people I wished I served with. They seemed wise, informed, and creative compared to the dull ignorance of the servile military culture I knew. I eventually joined the organization Iraq Veterans Against the War (I.V.A.W.).

Immersed in this environment and surrounded by like-minded peers of the Iraq War (which was escalating and getting uglier), I first made my uniform into paper at the invitation of the creators of The Combat Paper Project (http://www.combatpaper.org). At that time there were dozens of other veterans who had pulped their uniforms. The blank sheets, prints, and handmade books were stunningly beautiful, and it was hard to believe they originated from a military uniform. The process began by cutting the uniforms into small squares: the liberation of the rag. As I cut the uniform I had previously and painstakingly kept clean and pressed, the one that bore my name, rank, unit patch, and nation's flag, I half expected a belligerent First Sergeant to burst in and flip the table like Jesus to the money changers (McGrath, 2022). Together a small group of us told stories about our time in the military, as we transformed our uniforms into neat piles on the table. The cut-down rag was then fed into a Hollander beater and turned into pulp. The pulp was put into a vat, and I quickly formed it into sheets. The next morning, I eagerly peeled the dry sheets apart. At a large table I bound some of my sheets into a small journal (Figure 7.10) alongside others in the group. The process was complete. My uniform became a stack of handmade paper, and I became a papermaker.

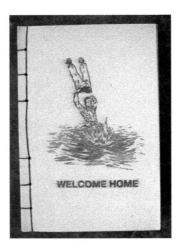

Figure 7.10 Homecoming.

It wasn't the army or the war that got me into papermaking. It was my reaction *to* the war that put me on the path to the vat. Pulping my uniform became a way for me to fight back against militarism (Figure 7.11). It sure felt like a better plan than throwing a rock through the windshield of my recruiter's Dodge Stratus. In the Bible, the Prophet Isaiah told the people to "beat their swords into plowshares ... and learn war no more" (English Standard Version Bible, 2016, Isaiah, 2:3–4). To that I would add: "they shall beat uniforms into pulp!"

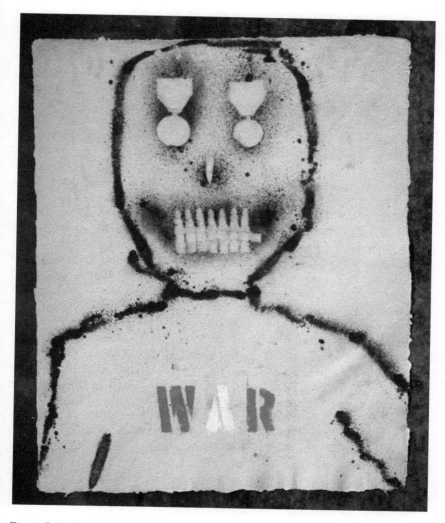

Figure 7.11 The Recruiters Came to My Middle School and All I Got Was This T-Shirt.

I pulped the last of my personal uniforms long ago. Now I work with several small groups of veterans making paper from military uniforms across the country through Frontline Arts (http://www.frontlinearts.org), Peace Paper Project (http://www.peacepaperproject.org), and Out of Step Press (http://www.outof-steppress.com). Usually, the workshop has been hosted by a university, veteran center, Veteran Affairs (V.A.) hospital, museum, or arts organization with participants from the military community. Veterans, active duty or reserve military, and their family members are the most common participants and are asked to bring a uniform to make into paper. Often, they will have brought a full duffle bag and donated what could not be pulped. I have slowly worked through this growing stockpile from facilitating these papermaking workshops.

On my handmade bookshelf sits a binder the size of a large photo album. In it is a collection of papers and small pieces of the uniform they were made from. The binder acts as a registry for the people I've worked with over the years. There are lots of greens and browns, with blue representing the Navy uniform. A pure white sheet shows the oldest uniform I've pulped. It came in the mail from an anonymous donor and a note that only explained "my father's 1940s Navy uniform." Presumably taken from the closet after the owner's death. Too sentimental to throw out. Too ordinary to keep. No return address was given.

Several sheets in the binder are called "memorial sheets," paper made from a uniform brought in by friends or family. Often their loved one had died, usually by suicide, killed in action, or in a mundane accident long after their service. Sometimes still showing blood and burn stains in the fibers. I keep a sheet and label it. It goes into the binder. Sometimes friends or other veterans turned artists joined us and made paper. Their uniforms went into the binder as well. Sometimes a uniform was long gone. Thrown into a dumpster or burn barrel. In these instances, a piece of clothing representing the veteran's service would be pulped as a stand-in for their military uniform. Perhaps baby clothes from a child born while on deployment, a T-shirt from a military unit reunion or association. I'm still waiting to make paper from a Space Force uniform. The binder could use some shiny silver or galactic purple among all the earthen hues.

Slowly I've acquired the skills and tools to make a book from scratch. I've made three poetry chapbooks by hand (Lewis, 2009; Lewis, 2012). Together these books tell my war stories. They illustrate my thoughts and experiences, show the scars, and keep alive the humor that many of us relied on to get through the war as human beings. I don't like my writing from ten years ago and I can hardly recognize the person who wrote them. Fortunately, handmade books tend to be very limited and the edition size very small. I've kept a few around. I am still amazed that they are out there somewhere in this world. A piece of war rag refuse hidden on a library shelf.

Even now, 20 years after the army, I can sit down at a sheet of paper and the stories and thoughts pour onto the page, often with the slightest encouragement of a writing prompt. Sometimes current events stir things up. It doesn't hurt to save the war in a box until later.

I continue to interact with a rapidly changing world through papermaking. A 2,000-year-old craft seems an odd way to communicate my objections to satellite-guided drone warfare or thermonuclear catastrophe. My own uniform gave me a platform to record my stories and thoughts. Many veterans lack this essential opportunity. In many ways pulping a uniform is a revolutionary act. The original item changes so profoundly and completely that it ceases to resemble or function as its former self. I think of the uniforms that turn into small flyers for parents to sign and legally opt-out their children's contact information for recruiters. The uniforms become prints sold at fundraisers for organizations devoted to fighting militarism. The uniforms turn into works of art that stimulate discussions among veterans and civilians. Sometimes it is after these discussions that minds are changed.

*

My Autoethnographic Research: Pulping My Late Father's T-shirts and Ties

Annie McFarland

Connections to Papermaking

My first papermaking memory came from a summer arts camp in Michigan when I was 12 years old. I remember taking recycled papers and using kitchen blenders to create small sheets of handmade paper. After returning to school in the Fall, I quickly forgot about this medium and focused more on academic matters and formal art classes. I pursued a Bachelor of Fine Arts in photography and graphic design and worked as a web and graphic designer after graduation. After short employment in Michigan's 2008 economy, the company I worked for closed and I was left searching for a new job. I started considering alternate career paths. I felt a strong desire to connect with others through art and creativity beyond the commercial realm.

During an online search, I came across an article about veterans using art to process and heal from post-traumatic stress disorder (P.T.S.D.) (McElveen, 2007). The use of the arts for healing was intriguing but also resonated with me because the military was an integrated component of my family when I was growing up. My father was a 6-year naval Vietnam veteran who later served in the U.S. Army Reserve for 25 years. This combined focus on the arts and veterans sparked my interest in art therapy. Within several weeks, I moved to Florida, applied to Florida State University's (F.S.U.) graduate art therapy program (http://arted.fsu.edu/programs/art-therapy), and was accepted the following year.

While attending F.S.U., I was able to explore a variety of media and therapeutic approaches with diverse populations in art therapy settings. However, my clinical interest continually returned to working with military veterans. In the spring of 2012, master papermaker Drew Matott and art therapist Gretchen Miller visited F.S.U. to present a lecture and interactive workshop on papermaking with veteran populations. I was thrilled to learn how papermaking could also use fabric and clothing. In contrast to the recycled papermaking process I encountered at summer camp, this method utilized a Hollander beater. This portable fiber processing unit ran on a small farm motor, which was powered by a wheel with ice skate-like blades. This broke down pieces of fabric into individual fibers, releasing the organic threads and transforming the raw material into paper pulp for creating sheets of handmade paper. The fabric was often an article of personal significance: a T-shirt someone used to wear, a uniform from military service, or even a baby blanket.

Matott and Miller also offered a hands-on workshop at the veteran's facility where I was completing my final practicum. Seeing veterans take their chosen clothing items and transform them into beautiful and expressive art pieces was an incredibly meaningful process. Witnessing the benefits of this therapeutic medium in action motivated me to focus my research studies on papermaking. My thesis project started with developing a veteran-centered curriculum guide for papermaking using personally significant fabrics. This became the basis for my doctoral dissertation. I also continued to help clients and artists work through trauma and grief through papermaking, including a 6-week international tour co-leading papermaking workshops in the U.K. and Germany with the Peace Paper Project.

During this time, I struggled with an intense personal loss of my own. On October 3, 2017, my father was diagnosed with an inoperable glioblastoma brain tumor, developed because of exposure to the chemical Agent Orange while serving in the Vietnam War. Over the course of six short weeks, his health declined rapidly. Three brain surgeries and an extended stay in the neuro-intensive care unit offered little hope to fight the fast growth of the tumor. He died on December 10, 2017.

As my family and I processed our collective grief, we began to sort through my father's possessions. We came across many personal belongings that documented a lifetime of lived experiences: business cards, books, photographs, tools, office supplies, and miscellaneous 1950s memorabilia. These items seemed to hold memory and connection to who he once was. I found myself wanting to preserve these articles, a haphazard collection of objects that also included many his ties and T-shirts (Figure 7.12). Looking back now, the obvious answer for the use of his clothing was to engage in papermaking. However, at that time, my art therapy research and practice focused on facilitating art-making experiences for others. Also, while I was comfortable helping others to process their grief, loss, and trauma, I wasn't ready to engage in that process myself.

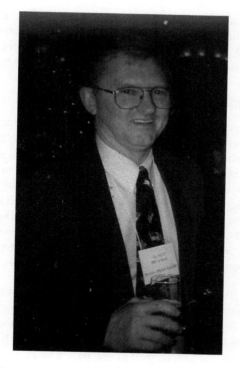

Figure 7.12 My father wearing one of his ties.

As time passed, my focus shifted to future job prospects in academia. I began a full-time university teaching position and simultaneously completed my doctoral dissertation research. My mind was occupied by professional and financial concerns, but I often found myself returning to that bag full of my father's clothing stashed away in the closet. In my university work, I began researching grant funding opportunities in art therapy and the visual arts. Through colleagues, I found out about the Myers Foundation Faculty Distinguished Research Award Program, which focused on arts-based projects and professional development. When reading about the opportunity for creative exploration and research through this grant, I immediately thought about exploring my own loss further to understand better the complexities and nuances of papermaking through an autoethnographic lens. I was finally ready to look at my own grief and loss to transform my father's clothing. I applied for the grant and was gratified to receive funding for my research.

I jumped right into papermaking and video-recorded the process from start to finish. It was difficult to think about each step in the moment, so reviewing videos and transcriptions were extremely helpful in understanding my own experiences from a third-person perspective. Engaging in this medium myself provided new realizations and allowed me to empathize with others participating in this method. Three steps within the papermaking process were especially illuminating: *selecting the fabric, cutting the fabric,* and *the final product itself.*

Selecting the Fabric

As I started gathering my father's ties and T-shirts, I was struck by the immediate emotional experience of selecting materials. Each item held a connection to a memory of my father: the ties he wore to work (Figure 7.13) and the T-shirts he wore around the house (Figure 7.14). Each one connected an abstract memory to a concrete, physical item. Selecting a few ties and T-shirts was a difficult emotional and cognitive task, but was lessened in impact because I had several items to choose from. I thought back to the clients I'd worked with who only had *one* article of clothing to use. How difficult their decision must have been: to part with a physical representation of an experience or memory knowing the papermaking process would ultimately destroy this remaining tangible connection to the past.

I found myself prioritizing and evaluating each item with a self-imposed ranking of importance. Color and symbols were most important for me when looking through his ties. Color also seemed to be associated with personality and memory. Which colors were "most" like him? I ultimately settled on several blue- and green-colored ties, as well as one with a small American flag pattern (Figure 7.15). When looking through his T-shirts, I considered color but also related to the level of wear. As white undershirts, some were new and some were well-worn, the latter being yellowed and faded. I connected the yellowed shirts as more representative of him because they'd been used over time. I correlated these items with a stronger connection to his physical presence. This experience

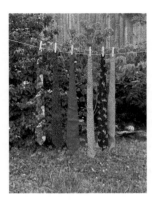

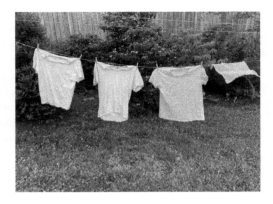

Figure 7.13 My father's ties.   *Figure 7.14* My father's T-shirts.

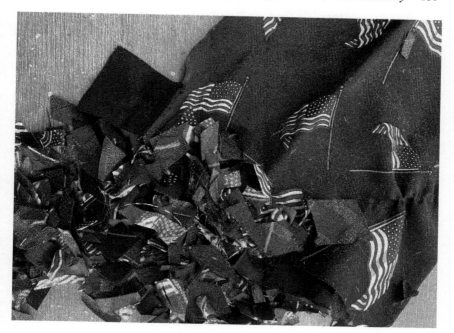

Figure 7.15 American flag tie details.

also provided insight into how my clients may have felt when thinking about how many times they'd worn a uniform. The more used it was, the more connected to memory and the past it may have held.

Cutting the Fabric

After the emotional task of selecting which fabrics to use, I was ready to cut and process the material. However, I was again surprised by the unexpected emotional and sensory-based nature of cutting the fibers. As I began deconstructing each item, I found every piece released an aroma specific to its wear. The ties (Figure 7.16) gave off a hint of starch and fabric softener; his T-shirts (Figure 7.17) smelled of the cedar cabinet where he stored his clothing along with a hint of perspiration from years of wear. Reviewing the video footage of this process, I talked about the preservation of memory and its relationship to physical connection. The smell of my father's shirts especially triggered questions for me about how many times he wore them. Where was he going? What events was he attending? Each whiff of item-specific smell seemed to generate reminiscence and connect our shared memories together. This experience helped me gain a greater understanding of the power of smell in relation to memory. It also reminded me of a time I attended a papermaking workshop where participants

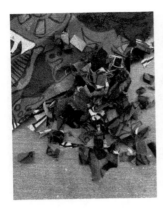 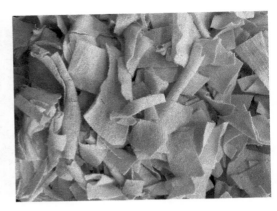

Figure 7.16 Pieces of ties.   *Figure 7.17* Pieces of T-shirts.

used donated naval uniforms. I vividly remembered the smell of diesel fuel as I began cutting the cloth. When cutting my father's clothing, however, the sensory experience was different. It was more intense. Through these objects, I made emotional connections to the lived experiences of my father.

Processing the Fibers and the Final Product

After cutting the fabric, I processed the fibers in my Hollander beater. I'd done this step many times before with clients and workshop participants. I assumed this portion of the papermaking process would be the most emotionally taxing. To my surprise, pulping the fiber and pulling sheets of wet paper was quite relaxing and felt intrinsically therapeutic. The sensory experiences within this step provided a grounding and soothing break from the emotionality of the previous steps. The water, being outside barefoot in the grass, and the breeze, all seemed to help me get into the flow and rhythm of pulling the sheets. I was able to pull, press, and hang 40 to 50 sheets of paper with relative ease (Figure 7.18).

As I looked at the visible fibers in every sheet, each one was different. Threads from my dad's ties were embedded throughout (Figure 7.19). The colors varied tremendously, and each sheet seemed to have its own unique configuration. My mind reflected on the metaphors present within this process. Every piece connected to a physical representation of him, his memory, and our lived experiences together. The paper's individuality made me think of the power of singular experiences and how all these memories added up to a lifetime of existence. The threads within the paper symbolized the interconnected fibers of relationship and memory.

As the entire papermaking process concluded, I had anxiety about how to use the paper. Like the resistance to pulping my father's clothing, I hesitated to "ruin" this material with a surface treatment that I wasn't satisfied with.

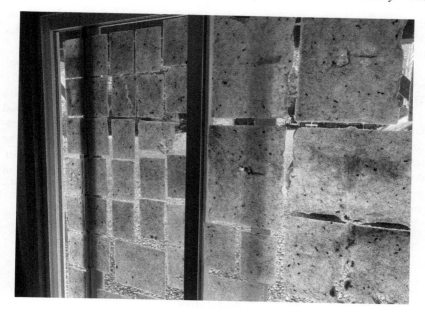

Figure 7.18 Paper **drying** on glass.

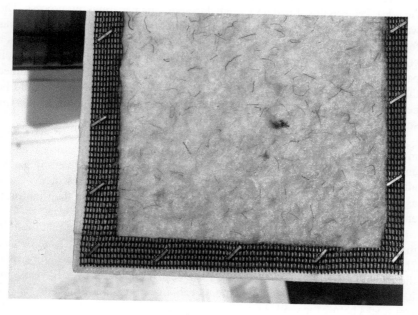

Figure 7.19 Fiber detail within the handmade paper.

Even though I created over 40 sheets, drawing or painting on them seemed too permanent. I felt myself wanting to preserve these papers, saving them for something special. I still have the papers, untouched, stacked safely in my office.

This mindset reminded me of the constant balance often discussed in art therapy: is it the *process* or the *product* which is most important? (Van Lith, 2015). Through my autoethnographic research, I've found value in *both*. The process was an emotional, and sometimes triggering, experience that must be approached with empathy and care. In turn, the art product itself was representative of a transformative, moving, and often poignant process toward healing and growth. The resulting product held so much more meaning than just a simple sheet of paper. As I progress forward in my own journey of healing, I plan to create portraits of my father printed on this paper for my family. This paper lives on, holding the memory of my father's life and his positive influence on those he touched.

*

Art Therapy Student to Art Therapist: Papermaking Lessons & Professional Practice

Rachel Mims

My first experience with papermaking was as a participant in a Peace Paper Project workshop on campus at Florida State University (F.S.U.) (http://www.fsu.edu). Prior to this, I had no knowledge about the papermaking process. The workshop took place early in my first semester as a graduate student and was for F.S.U.'s Collegiate Veterans Association (C.V.A.) (McMackin, 2021). As a veteran and art therapy student, I encouraged other student veterans to participate. My peers were reluctant to agree, but I described the process and explained that it could be a valuable experience. While I knew the workshop would be beneficial to the other participants, I erroneously assumed that, as an art therapy student, it would not affect me in the same way.

One of the first things we did during the workshop was cut up one of our military uniforms. Although I knew that I would never wear my uniform again, and it would likely just sit in storage if I kept it, I was hesitant to cut it up. We all had a strong emotional attachment to our uniforms; they represented a major aspect of our identity. Some participants were not able to cut up their uniforms and, instead, they used donated uniforms from their branch of service.

My emotions about my uniform were somewhat tied to the fact that I left the military after an injury that I never fully recovered from. I went from being a "high speed, squared away" soldier to "worthless" in the eyes of the army. Even though this was a difficult experience, I had been a soldier for over 10 years, and it was a huge part of my identity. I thought about cutting up my uniform for several weeks before the workshop, wondering, "can I really cut it up?" Eventually, I concluded that because of my disability I would never wear my uniform again and it was okay to cut it up. When interviewed about this part of the experience, I was brought to tears (Matott, 2016).

Looking back at the papermaking process, I realize that I compartmentalized my emotions during the workshop. I do not remember feeling emotional during the pulping process. Instead, I focused on learning how to make paper from the pulp. After I got the process down, I began to experiment with using more than one color of paper and with different images.

As the group progressed through the papermaking process, I began to think about what the process meant to me, and the paper I was making began to sig-nify my transition from military life to civilian life. I created several pieces with a mix of light gray uniform paper and paper made from an F.S.U. T-shirt that was garnet. I also pulp printed Figure 7.20 on this paper of a PATRIOT mis-sile launcher, the vehicle I drove and operated while in the military. This paper represented still being enmeshed in military culture while also doing my best to move toward the life I had dreamed about for several years. I never felt like my transition was especially difficult but looking back I realized this was because I was lucky enough to be in such a supportive environment. At F.S.U. I had the support of other student veterans, my art therapy classmates, the veteran's center, and the art therapy program staff. I probably would have struggled much more without these people in my life.

As part of the workshop, F.S.U. allowed us to pick our favorite piece and they had it framed for exhibition. Having Figure 7.20 framed helped me *not* regret cutting up my uniform because I could proudly display it on my wall instead of

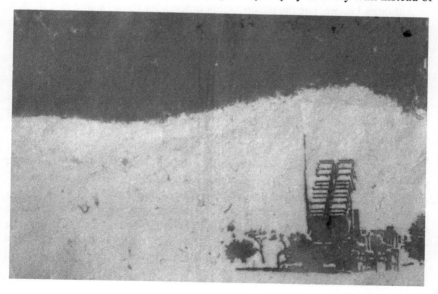

Figure 7.20 Amalgam. Handmade paper from my military uniform and a school T-shirt.

it being hidden in storage. The image has been hanging in my living room since the day I received it. It is still one of my favorite pieces out of all the art I have made.

The group from the papermaking workshop showed our art at the annual Veterans Film Festival held by F.S.U. every November. This gave us the opportunity to talk about our work with others. Later we displayed our pieces at the main library on campus. Again, we were afforded the opportunity to discuss our work and the papermaking experience with the public. During the library exhibit opening, a fellow participant stated that this process allowed him to take what was inside of him and put it outside.

This experience changed me as a person as it allowed me to process complicated emotions during a time of major change, and it helped me establish a bond with the other workshop participants. It also helped me realize how my future clients could feel if they went through this process. I think the experience made me a better therapist and I suggest being a participant to anyone who has the opportunity.

My second papermaking experience was two years later at another workshop held for veterans at F.S.U. I had recently graduated but was asked to come back and serve as the art therapist for this workshop. Being the therapist at the workshop was completely different. This time around, I was focused on the experience of others instead of my own experience. It was very moving to see the connections others had to their military service and how they were honoring that experience through papermaking.

Although I appreciate the papermaking process for the art that it is, I think it is the personal significance of the cloth used that made these workshops so powerful. Adding a personal image to our paper also enhanced the impact. Lastly, participating as a group greatly impacted our relationships by bonding us. Prior to participating in the workshop, I had not felt connected to any of the veterans in the C.V.A. because we had only just met and did not know each other well. During this workshop, we shared stories about our time in the military and had the opportunity to learn about each other's current life as well. When I returned to F.S.U. to participate in the workshop as an art therapist, I did not know the participants as most of them were new students who had started school after I graduated. Again, the workshop afforded me the opportunity to learn more about their past experiences as well as the hopes and goals of those who were participating. These participants were able to bond as a group too.

My experiences with papermaking have demonstrated to me the therapeutic benefit of this process. It is something I know can help people heal from past trauma and grief, and can aid in major life transitions. This is something I hope to do with my clients moving forward so that they too can have this powerful and healing experience.

*

When the Pulp Dries: Claiming the Self through Paper Exhibitions

Erin Mooney-Simkus

At the Veterans Administration (V.A.) hospital where I worked as an art therapist, my program was lucky enough to have the space and support to regularly offer veteran papermaking workshops facilitated by Peace Paper Project (Matott & Miller, 2020). They introduced veterans to the papermaking process, different media, and art processes, as well as the idea of art as a transformative experience. Some veterans participated many times over the years, as they developed their own papermaking process and deepened their art experience. The veterans often asked when they could make paper again.

The deconstruction of the uniform, the noise of the Hollander beater, and the sensory experience of the water were all outside the participants' everyday encounters. The veterans were often skeptical of the process and unsure about their abilities to create when they began it. However, papermaking was immediately engaging and accessible. This hesitation quickly shifted and became a source of pride and creative energy.

Papermaking also provided a unique opportunity to come together in a community and share in an art process that engaged cognitive, symbolic, affective, perceptual, and kinesthetic expressions (Hinz, 2009). Participants created meaningful work to process their inner experiences in a space designed to support connections with themselves and others. The veterans shared stories about their time in the service, where they were stationed, and where they were currently.

During the workshop's first couple of years, I also worked in the hospital's inpatient psychiatric unit. I was not able to bring the hands-on papermaking process into that space due to safety constraints. However, I still wanted to share papermaking with these veterans. This was accomplished by using pre-made paper, fabricated from military uniforms. I brought stacks of this handmade paper to my inpatient art therapy groups and described its origin, explaining in detail the process of papermaking, the materials, and methods that were used, as well as how this art-making was an opportunity to create internal and external change and understanding.

My intention was that this group could connect with the process and concept even though they didn't necessarily have an opportunity to create the paper themselves. Much of my personal reflection artwork and process shared within my groups at this time were based on mandalas. I encouraged participants to create a design or image inside a circle on the handmade paper. Ideas about art as a form of active meditation, a place to quiet the mind, connect with oneself, and a way to focus on small tasks within a contained space were introduced.

Then one year, in celebration of Veterans Day, the hospital hosted a Veteran Art Exhibition and a papermaking demonstration in the atrium outside the cafeteria. The display featured some of the veterans' mandalas from the inpatient unit. In this exhibition space, veterans interacted with their artwork, had an opportunity to see the papermaking process, and created their own paper if they chose to do so. The exhibition brought the healing and transformative process of art and papermaking outside of the usual art therapy group spaces and into the communal areas within the hospital. This shift valued sharing one's experience with peers and staff who may not have typically interacted with the art therapy process.

As an art therapist, I was mindful of the intentions of displaying veteran artwork. I ensured the art exhibition focused on the positive impact of the creative process and viewers observing this narrative. It is important to note, that I always gave the veterans free choice about how to display their artwork, with no pressure to participate, and I supported veterans who chose to display their work anonymously. I also discussed the implications of displaying one's art and how deciding to exhibit work can invite comments from strangers about a deeply personal process (American Art Therapy Association, 2013; Vick, 2011). Conversely, the display provided an opportunity for the veterans who participated to see themselves in relation to one another or in contrast to others' experiences.

The concept of displaying artwork at V.A. hospitals has a long history of pride and honor due to the Veterans Creative Arts Festival (http://www/creativeartsfestival.va.gov), an annual art competition where veterans have competed locally and then nationally in a variety of art, drama, dance, music, and creative writing categories (U.S. Department of Veterans Affairs, 2021). This celebration has also focused on the healing power of arts engagement, including creative expressions that may or may not have been created within a therapeutic relationship. The quality of the finished pieces was the primary focus of this competition. In contrast, the hospital's Veterans Day art exhibit focused on the process and the veterans' emotional experiences. There was less regard for creating an aesthetic product. The pride of sharing the work and the veterans' personal stories was a different type of recognition.

A couple of years after the Veterans Day Exhibition, there was an initiative at the hospital to install a Healing Arts Gallery. The idea was to provide a dedicated space where the veterans could display their artwork, as well as advocate for veterans and inform viewers about the diversity of the veteran experience. In addition, displaying art that was created in a therapeutic environment highlighted the value and impact of the creative process and its ability to promote growth and healing, a foundation of art therapy. There was a distinct type of knowing that came with experiencing the visible emotional effect and exploration of another's artwork. It's not a verbal explanation with facts and data. It was a sharing of one's "felt" sense, which the viewer acknowledged and interacted with non-verbally and then processed how this encounter shaped and affected them. When expressed and identified, this awareness could be seen by the self and others.

All these exhibitions featured and displayed art from the papermaking workshops and invited the veterans to create imagery communicating their experiences. The exhibits authentically told the veterans' stories of their time in the military outside of their service. The integration and understanding of the art's emotion and its symbolism encouraged viewers to also feel these expressions. Everyone within the hospital community who viewed these exhibits over the years has had an opportunity to learn more about the veteran experience. This interaction of increased awareness can create a shift in our worldview. When the life stories of others have an impact on us, this narrative becomes an avenue for change in our communities and connections to each other.

*

Immigration, Advocacy, and Papermaking

Yaslin M. Torres-Peña

I am a proud daughter of Mexican immigrants. Both of my parents (Figure 7.21) migrated to the United States from Mexico to give their families back home a better life and to build a family here. My father crossed the Tijuana and California border by foot a total of eight times, traveling about 1,640 miles before he began his life in the U.S. and started a family in Los Angeles, California. He walked across the desert in the heat with the dream of providing a better life for his family. I often find myself thinking, "Would I have been able to make that journey eight times?" I also think about how different my life would be if my dad didn't keep trying to make his dream come true.

My father's story was tough. The first couple of times my dad crossed, he shared that he had just enough money to make the journey so when he got *al otro lado* [to the other side] he went right to work in the orchards of California. He slept in the orchards that were the furthest away from the light so he could "comfortably" build a fire when there was space, or where he could at least sleep for a couple of hours. He said he heard the coyotes howling. Although it was scary to hear them so close, it was better than the days he heard *MMIIGGRAAA!*, a slang term that alerted him to the U.S. Immigration and Customs Enforcement (I.C.E.) or immigration police. There were several times my dad would lay flat in the tall grass for days because the fear of being taken was so high. For dinner, he went to the closest convenience store, and for weeks he bought raw eggs to eat and drank Coke. After working day and night to save enough money to start building a real home, he did. He brought his wife over with him and started a family.

My family lived in an area with high poverty and gang violence in Los Angeles, so my father chose to move us to Moses Lake, Washington. I.C.E. called on my family at least three times during the first couple of years we lived in Moses Lake. When we were out in the streets, there were racial slurs. My dad said that he would rather endure the pain of the comments than see his kids be endangered by the violence in Los Angeles.

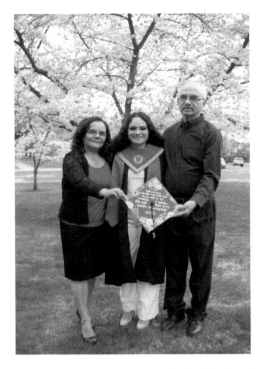

Figure 7.21 Left to right: Maria (my mom), me, and Maurilio (my dad). *Los amo papis.*

My mother was fortunate enough to have received a visa in Mexico and entered the U.S. legally. When she arrived in Moses Lake, she went straight to work in packaging warehouses and then, eventually, at a very prominent potato company where she worked for over eight years. After marrying my dad, she gained U.S. residency. My mother was always so eager to learn and get an education, since she was not able to in Mexico. She dedicated herself to getting an education. She also had the dream of working as an office assistant, so she applied to Big Bend Community College. She studied countless nights to earn her G.E.D. (General Educational Diploma), which she completed in English, despite the language barrier. She didn't stop there. She continued her education in business management. In 2008 I had the greatest honor of seeing my mother walk the stage and receive her diploma. She is a constant reminder of why I cannot give up.

My dad always dreamed about his kids succeeding in this land of opportunities and reaching higher education. All five of his kids have received bachelor's degrees. From the time I can remember I had always said I wanted to be a doctor. As I grew older, I learned how hard that was. I worked extremely hard throughout high school to get into a 4-year university. My goal was to attend Baylor School of Medicine and become a Physician Assistant. I decided to pursue a Bachelor of Science in Biology at Washington State University Tri-Cities (W.S.U. T.C.) (http://wsu.edu). As a first-generation student, my parents couldn't provide guidance because of their limited experience, so I had to seek my own opportunities. My grade point average (G.P.A.) suffered and was nowhere near what I expected of myself. As a first-generation Mexican-American there was an unspoken pressure to become a doctor, lawyer, or engineer. It was like having those titles proved the worth of our families here in the U.S. I realized I wasn't chasing my dream, but I was chasing my family's dream. But later that changed.

After my second year at W.S.U. T.C., I became involved with the Dreamers Club (http://tricities-wsu.presence.io/organization/dreamers-club) and held the positions of treasurer and then president (Washington State University, 2021). The Dreamers Club strived for the educational, cultural, social, economic, and political representation of our undocumented community. On-campus, we held immigration information sessions, cultural celebrations, and, most importantly a bilingual multicultural graduation. This was where I discovered my passion for advocacy. I spent most of my time within the club pushing for better representation and resources for Latinx students, specifically those who were undocumented. Although I am not undocumented and will never know what this feels like, *yo luchaba para mi familia* [I fought for my family]. I related to my peers in this student community, regardless of their immigration status because of our culture and the shared fear of a loved one's deportation.

2018 was when I was first introduced to papermaking and realized how much meaning this project could have for our group. This event was described as an opportunity for students to experience art as therapy. As a club on campus, we were invited to share our stories and experience of what our labor could make. When the process was first demonstrated my initial reaction was that it was cool but, after making paper with a piece of clothing that was personally meaningful, it was amazing. Everyone either had worked or had a loved one who worked in the fields, so we all chose to pulp a shirt that was worn during this time. I personally used someone's shirt who was very special to me and who I knew had worked hard to have everything he currently had. When I was cutting up his shirt, I was not just thinking about him, but I was also thinking about my entire family who had given this country their all. They worked day and night, and missed holidays, birthdays, or important events because this country depended on the work of our immigrant families. The eight times it took my dad to cross, the language discrimination my mom encountered, and all the blood, sweat, and tears were now a piece of paper. During this year President Trump was persistent about building a wall between the U.S. and Mexico (U.S.A. Today, 2017) so I decided that one of the sheets would be stenciled with a brick wall and the words "WE BELONG HERE." We do, we do belong here.

During my third year at W.S.U. T.C. in 2019, the campus had another papermaking workshop with Peace Paper Project. This time, I chose a piece of clothing to signify the career change I wanted to make. I was still a biology major struggling mentally through school in a field I enjoyed but knew was not what I wanted to do. When I cut up my shirt and made my paper, I truly found my passion.

On my very first sheet, I **pulp printed** two hands reaching for each other with the world in the middle (Figure 7.22). Although the image didn't mean much to me then, now I see that the hands reaching for the world symbolized that the world was in my hands. I can choose what I want to change, and am worthy of making my own choices, not those of society (Figure 7.23). Later that year I registered for history and English, two classes completely out of my major. I enjoyed my history class so much that in my fourth year I changed my major to political science.

My family has always shown me the value of persistence and chasing your dreams. I can now say with confidence that my dream career is to serve the people, and I am pursuing this goal. My extended family's legal status and my

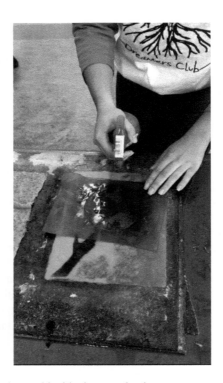

Figure 7.22 Printing the world with pigmented pulp.

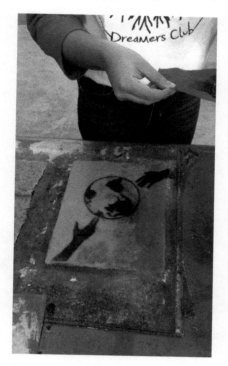

Figure 7.23 You are the author of your own story.

parents' background have motivated me to educate and build support for the undocumented and Latinx communities. One day I wish to open a center in Moses Lake that will serve as a safe space with resources for immigrant students and entire families. I want all Black, Indigenous, and People of Color (B.I.P.O.C.) immigrant families to feel like the world is also at the tips of their fingers and everything they dreamed about is attainable regardless of their status (Figure 7.24).

Recently, I was working with undocumented farmworkers on the east side of Washington as an Emergency Relief organizer. My job was to help give farmworkers a voice: a voice my parents, family, and community members never had. That is why I have chosen to tell our story.

Often when I first thought of my family's work, it was about the crops or packaging companies, not a sheet of handmade paper. A piece of paper seems so simple. Yet its contents, fibers, and art made with the paper gives people the opportunity to tell their stories …. just as I have been able to do here.

*

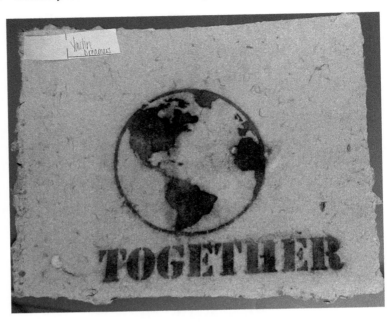

Figure 7.24 Pulp print of the world on green paper.

Transformation in Papermaking: When Content Mirrors Process

Denise R. Wolf

Papermaking has been called a double process (Ash, 2017): one that both destroys and creates, resulting in a tangible manifestation of change. Innate kinesthetic-sensory qualities invite opportunities for sensory-based integration (Hinz, 2020). Both the content and process of papermaking mirror the way the consequences of trauma are ameliorated.

The act of making paper out of a litany of substrate options holds an incredible amount of potential, but the most profound component to me is the concept that you are engaging in a creative process to create a new surface, a blank slate, tabula rasa, and the feeling of starting over.

(Boone, 2021 para. 1)

Through my own clinical practice, I have come to identify two core concepts of change implicit in trauma recovery. A client must ask and identify the answers to the following two inquiries: who am I now that this event has happened and what is this world that such an event can take place in it? (Wolf & King, 2021). The word trauma itself is hypothesized to have come from the Latin *tere*, to rub, thresh, grind, or wear away (Trauma, 2020). Art therapists use the creative process as a "paradigm of everyday experiences" (Rubin, 2011, p. 88; McNiff,

1998). The way we use art materials and methods is specialized (King, 2016). Papermaking is a mirrored process of destruction and reformation. It culminates in an externalized and often aesthetically pleasing product that has a new meaning and purpose. Fundamental to papermaking is a scaffolded, iterative process, well suited to treat trauma (Kay & Wolf, 2017).

Trauma theorist and psychiatrist Bruce Perry (2009) identified the "Six Rs" as integral in trauma recovery work and these can be found embedded in the papermaking process. According to Perry, therapy must contain elements of *rhythm* and *repetition*, and be *relational, relevant, respectful,* and *rewarding. Rhythmic* encounters resonate with neural patterns that assist in the regulation of the autonomic nervous system, creating a sense of calm (Perry, 2009). Cadenced movements are fundamentally embedded in papermaking processes. Trauma is stored in the body and can be reworked and released through movement and regulatory stimulation (Van der Kolk, 2014). Dipping the mould and deckle into a vat of pulp also requires a rhythmic motion so that the pulp or slurry is evenly distributed on the screen. This process requires that the maker **shake** the deckle forward and backward, side to side, to help the fibers interlock. There is *repetition* in cutting or tearing cloth, paper, or fibers to create pulp, in pulling sheets of paper, and in the stacking of wet sheets between **linters** and cardboard. Perry identifies repetition in trauma therapy as encounters that are predictable and repeated over time. This fosters safety, familiarity, and a sense of agency. In a materials and processes graduate art therapy class, one of my students observed that, "engaging in the papermaking process by following repetitive steps may create a sense of control and independence over one's life" (Fourney, 2021). Interpersonal or *relational* encounters transpire through a therapeutic alliance with the facilitator, as well as other participants in the papermaking studio. The creation of stations offers participants opportunities for peer problem-solving and interpersonal interaction (Wolf, 2018). The therapist bears witness to the deconstructed state, holding space for the emergence of an enduring state of strength, as symbolized in the result.

By creating paper from deconstructed materials that hold personal meaning to the creator, the process develops *relevance*. Both my students and clients have used parts of love letters, hate letters, old tests, pregnancy test instructions, and discharge paperwork, thereby deconstructing, transforming, and then birthing something new. Allen, a graduate art therapy student commented, "Being able to see and feel a tangible, creative product (Figure 7.25) gave me a new sense of meaning in this process" (2021, para. 1).

Processes that are *respectful* of the participant are enacted through the facilitator's provision of safety and autonomy. The primary functions of the facilitator are to control structure, media, and roles (Rubin, 2020). Graduate student Jessica (Paige, 2021, para. 4) remarked:

The process gives back a lot of control to the client. It allows for them to personally reframe an experience or an idea by tearing it down to shreds and building it back up in a way that benefits them. It is reframing their narrative.

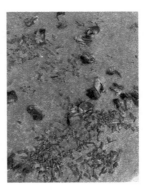

Figure 7.25 Paper in process.

The finished product is a tangible, tactile, and functional object or relic that was not in existence previously, a literal and symbolic *reward*. The finished sheet(s) of paper is a visual representation of the process, a physical embodiment of renewal (Hinz, 2020). Matott and Miller offer the succinct summary that, at its core, papermaking requires "purposeful, concrete and repetitive steps to safely engage" (2020, p. 312).

What follows is an exploration of my own clinical failure with handmade paper. Kramer (1986) considers the disclosure of therapist failure as an imperative part of clinical development. I affectionately think of this story as *Misadventures in Papermaking*. I was a novice art therapist working in residential treatment with adolescents. Many of these teens had experienced complex interpersonal trauma, such as physical and/or sexual abuse, residing in a dangerous neighborhood, placement in multiple foster homes, or exposure to domestic violence. Hand papermaking was an ongoing interest of mine, and I was looking forward to bringing this practice to the group. Beginning with a demonstration followed by separating and labeling each person's pulp, I set the teens to the task at stations placed around the room (Canto et al., 2015). I felt that I had prepared sufficiently. The noise level began to steadily rise as the adolescents responded to the kinesthetic-sensory experiences of interacting with cold slurry in large vats. *Chatter. Swish. Whizz.* The pulp began to soar across the room in gloopy clumps. *Splat. Shriek.* "There was a lot of screaming and yelling and crying, and that was just from me" (Wolf, 2018, p. 71). *Stop! Clean up, art therapy group is OVER!* I essentially kicked the members out of the studio, ending the group early. Renouncing any responsibility, I admonished them for their regressive and childish behaviors. Angrily, I began to clean up. As I wiped pulp from the walls, it occurred to me that *I* had failed. I had overlooked the necessity of creating a safe, structured, and scaffolded invitation to papermaking. Mostly what I had done was offer the group members a symbolic tub of dysregulated feelings

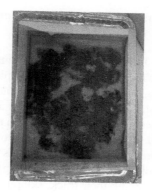

Figure 7.26 Mould and deckle.

and disenfranchised experiences, telling them to take a pulpy dive into chaos and discomfort. Some participants metaphorically plunged in headfirst, while others ran the gamut between hesitancy and an unequivocal refusal to engage at all. Sifting through and reforming my own mess, breaking it down, and putting it back together, allowed me a way to reframe my own "papermaking fail." I came to a new understanding. In the group the following week, I provided increased structure, papermaking stations, clear roles (*relational*), and, perhaps most importantly, an apology (*respectful* and *relevant*). The participants had opportunities to benefit from all of Perry's Six Rs (2009). The external structure of the group became the deckle and frame, containing the pulpy emotions! In response to a graduate class experiential (Figure 7.26), a student remarked, "Using the materials required to complete this process may offer boundaries to contain chaotic feelings and thinking" (Fourney, 2021).

Rankanen (2014) states that "the unpleasant experiences of facing negative emotions or thoughts foster constructive therapeutic change when the experience is integrated with emerging self-reflection and insights" (p. 203). This is yet another mirror of the papermaking process itself, one of transformation towards a tangible product and utility. Brandstrup, Miller, and Potash (2019) noted that the sharing of art therapy failures can result in enhanced professional insight and strengthen future relationships with clients. The voices of artists, teachers, and therapists are vital in art therapy education and practice potential. They can offer insights that are not often actualized in education or research. "Transformation can take place through reworking, revising, reframing, adjusting, or altering – all processes that hold symbolic value and thus have unique therapeutic potential" (Leone, 2020, p. 17). Although Leone was speaking about the use of ceramics in art therapy, the same holds true for the transformative processes inherent in papermaking.

*

Papermaking and the Process of Returning Home

Eli Wright

It was a brutally hot day in Ramadi during the summer of 2004. A few of us medics were sitting inside the Battalion Aid Station playing a video game while trying to escape the stifling desert heat. Just outside our door, a Humvee skidded to a halt in a cloud of dust. A panicked soldier burst inside, yelling "We need a medic!" One team member was already grabbing an aid bag, while I grabbed a litter and a pair of trauma scissors. We ran outside to the open rear door of the truck to see a pale, terrified young man holding his bloody leg, screaming in agony. One of the other soldiers blurted out something about a rocket-propelled grenade (R.P.G.) barely missing their truck, skipping across the pavement directly underneath the vehicle, and hitting this soldier who was taking cover from the ambush.

Miraculously, the R.P.G. didn't explode, but it hit him directly in the shin, nearly severing his right leg below the knee. As I assessed the damage and began cutting away his desert camouflage trousers, he grabbed at my scissors, pleading with me, "PLEASE don't let my leg fall off, Doc!" I stopped cutting, looked up at his gray, sweaty face, and assured him in my calmest voice as he began to lose consciousness, "Don't worry brother, I got you."

We carried the soldier inside our aid station, stopped the bleeding, established intravenous (I.V.) lines, bandaged, splinted, and stabilized his leg for transport, then sent him on the MedEvac helicopter to the surgical hospital in Baghdad. Afterward, we went back inside, cleaned up all the blood, and resumed playing our video game. It was just another day in the Iraq War, like so many others. But I'll never forget the look of terror in his eyes as I cut his pants away to expose that mangled mess of shattered bone and shredded muscle while lying to him that everything was going to be ok. I knew he wouldn't keep that leg, but we did our best to salvage it anyway.

A few years later, in the summer of 2007, an army buddy I was stationed with at Fort Drum, New York, invited me to a small art studio a few hours away in the basement of an old factory building in Burlington, Vermont. He said there were some veterans there who made paper out of their military uniforms and who also happened to be fellow members of the organization Iraq Veterans Against the War (I.V.A.W.). I knew that I had to go to see what was going on. I grabbed one of my old uniforms, went A.W.O.L. for the weekend, and showed up with my buddy at the Green Door Studio. I asked if they could turn my uniform into paper and they said, "no," but they would teach me how to do it myself and then handed me a pair of scissors.

One of the first lessons I learned in training as a combat medic was that to treat a wound, I had to completely expose it. All that body armor and camouflage, which were meant to shield and conceal us from danger, were just getting in the way once the blood started to flow. The first time I took those scissors to my own uniform, I suddenly understood how my wounds had been hidden since I came home. Once I began to cut, a flood of horrible memories and complicated emotions were suddenly unleashed, and I didn't have adequate language to describe them. I hadn't thought much about that soldier in Ramadi since the incident happened, but as I meticulously deconstructed each seam, I remembered hastily cutting his uniform off to assess his wounds. In that moment, I felt a profound connection to that young man whose name I never even knew. He was just one of many casualties I had cared for during my deployment to Iraq, and many more after I came back stateside. I had treated so many people's trauma that I became desensitized to my own because of that constant exposure. Like so many service members and veterans, I self-medicated with alcohol and pills to cope with the chronic physical and emotional pain of my experiences. The first time I gathered with other veterans to cut uniforms up together, I discovered an escape from that destructive abyss. That was the moment I became a papermaker, and I was hooked.

I continued to show up at the Green Door Studio every chance I had, and then, in 2008, I was medically retired from the army due to injuries I sustained while deployed. With nowhere else to go, I packed up my remaining uniforms and a few other belongings in my car and went back to Burlington. I was so grateful to have found a new community that shared a common interest, and I was determined to learn everything I could about the history and craft of papermaking.

During those early years of the Combat Paper Project, the most significant factor that connected many of us together was the collaborative, community-focused aspect of papermaking as a group. The process was naturally related to the teamwork-focused culture of the military. Papermaking contains many aspects of ritual and tradition in its lineage, two traits that also factor strongly in military culture. I quickly began to understand how militarism was deeply imbued throughout paper's entire historical journey, from its origins in ancient China, along the Silk Road trade routes through central Asia, from wars in Samarkand to Baghdad, across northern Africa into Europe and beyond (Bloom, 2001).

Discovering these connections with fellow veterans and this shared history that permeated across time and distance was lifesaving. Who knew we could take old, dirty, blood-stained rags that carried all these dark memories embedded within their fibers, and transform them into something positive? The inherent poetry of the process quickly found a home written on those empty pages we had produced from the fibers of our pasts. The indelible images burned in our brains could finally find somewhere else to live outside of those confines. One night in the studio, while making a large sheet of paper from black pulp, but unsure of what to do with it, I noticed a bucket full of red pulp sitting in a corner. Without much thought, I grabbed a large scoopful of the red pulp and violently flung it at the black sheet, creating what appeared to be a gaping, bleeding wound near the center of the composition (Figure 7.27). I became interested in the potential for paper to mimic certain qualities of human anatomy, such as its tendency

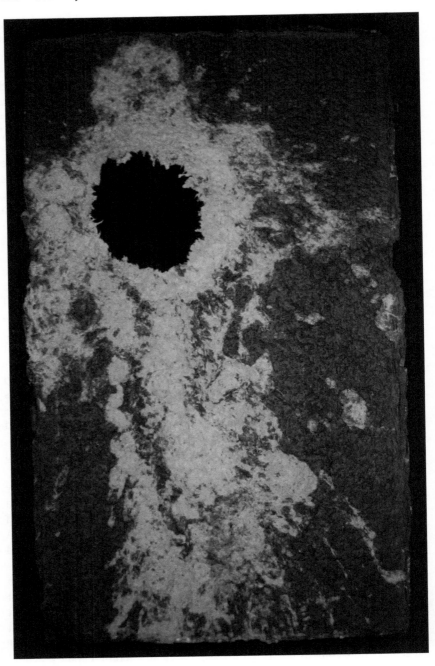

Figure 7.27 Open Wound.

to stretch and wrinkle like skin. I began to explore paper as a metaphor for the body, with its dual nature of durability and fragility, and its capacity to be sculpted and formed to mimic muscle and viscera.

Externalizing inner trauma became a key component of the process. It felt crucial to impart a sense of shared responsibility upon our fellow countrymen for the suffering and destruction we had caused in Iraq and elsewhere and for the pain we were enduring because of those conflicts. It was as much about protest as it was about self-exploration. We were furiously productive back then, tearing through countless uniforms from every branch and era of service, producing thousands of sheets of paper, drinking copious amounts of beer, and disturbing the neighbors with loud music late into the night. Eventually it became clear that this creative process must be shared far and wide. It was much too important to keep to ourselves, so we hit the road, and a new adventure began. The more I learned, the more I realized that those papermaking workshops we developed were merely another iteration in a long line of artists and elders who had already done similar work. For example, I was heavily inspired by Dr. Eric Avery's work with patients living with HIV/AIDS and other infectious diseases (Avery, 2004). I also discovered the profoundly influential work John Risseeuw was doing with victims of landmines (Risseeuw, 2011). And certainly, without World War II veteran Douglass Howell's essential experimentation and contributions to handmade paper upon returning home from that war (Barron & Gosin, n.d.), I wouldn't even be writing this essay. Throughout much of the history of this craft, many practitioners have understood the significance of emblematic fibers and their incredibly impactful storytelling potential. Our mission couldn't be clearer.

When I first enlisted in the army in the immediate aftermath of 9/11, my intention (however misguided) was to help others by any means available. In practice, that included everything from providing care under fire in combat, to driving an ambulance, feeding, and bathing wounded troops at Walter Reed Army Medical Center, and ultimately, marching and organizing to bring the troops home to prevent further unnecessary pain and suffering. When I discovered the inherent therapeutic nature of making paper from symbolically significant articles of clothing, a whole new world of possibility opened. When my military service ended, I inadvertently discovered this other way to continue serving and assisting others with their own struggles. The significance of witnessing all these connections helped me understand my place in the world in a whole new way, at a time when I was utterly lost and searching for direction and purpose. Like new synaptic pathways forming in a traumatically injured brain, we all worked together to find new detours back to collect the broken pieces of ourselves we'd lost along the way. Although I could no longer work as a combat medic or an emergency medical technician (E.M.T.), I found that I could still do meaningful work that focused on that same essential mission – to help relieve others of their suffering. In doing so, I began my own healing process. This was one of the most liberating experiences I've continued to carry with me today, after more than 15 years of doing this work.

Traumatic experiences have a tendency of fracturing our sense of time and space. The act of cutting rag, pulling sheets, couching them onto felt, and repeating the process ad infinitum can be a tremendously calming and meditative practice. The sounds of ripping fabric and dripping water, and the feel of the wet pulp running between one's fingers in the vat are rich sensory experiences that can counteract symptoms of anxiety and depression in many beneficial ways. I have witnessed so many veterans enter the room, practically crawling out of their skin with anxiety, or nearly catatonic with depression, yet within hours, they're sharing stories with other participants, connecting the dots between their individual and collective experiences, sometimes crying, always laughing, and momentarily transformed back to *themselves* again. In those moments, there is hardly any separation between participant and instructor, where empathy and solidarity are crucial to making the process work.

As the work continues, the community has grown and evolved in many ways. Peace Paper Project, Frontline Arts, Out of Step Press, and other affiliated endeavors such as Warrior Writers, have adapted to carry on the community-focused collaborations and traditions that have been the lifeblood of this community since its inception in 2007. In 2011, David Keefe and I co-founded Frontline Arts. As an instructor, I've primarily focused my efforts on working with active-duty service members at military hospitals. Additionally, I've had the privilege of teaching many workshops at colleges and universities, arts festivals, and other venues such as Haystack Mountain School of Crafts and the Robert C. Williams Museum of Papermaking. I continue to develop my individual art practice, working in a variety of mixed-media printmaking. I am always experimenting and trying to discover new ways of understanding paper and its revolutionary history. In 2017, I and a few other veteran papermakers embarked on an intensive collaboration with filmmaker Talia Lugacy to develop the award-winning film *This Is Not a War Story* (http://www.acousticfilms.com), which prominently featured the papermaking process and how it is utilized as a means of intergenerational community-building among veterans struggling with the specter of suicide.

In the summer of 2020, I began working on a small homestead in rural New York, which will include a paper mill and guest cabin to host the next generation of young veterans who may find themselves on the journey of discovering paper. When I reflect on years of papermaking's history and how this simple, yet durable medium has faithfully carried the stories and images we've all imparted upon its surface, I always find myself looking deeper, beneath the surface, to consider the stories embedded between those fibers that bind us together. Perhaps one day we may learn to use paper solely as a medium for love letters and creative art, rather than declarations of war and suicide notes.

*

References

Allen, E. (2021). *Papermaking, transformation, and meaning making.* Unpublished manuscript. Drexel University.

American Art Therapy Association. (2013). Ethical principles for art therapists [Exhibition of Client Artwork]. https://arttherapy.org/wp-content/uploads/2017/06/Ethical-Principles-for-Art-Therapists.pdf.

Ash, J. (2017). The things paper carries: The combat paper project. *Art in Print, 6*(5), 11–15.

Avery, E. (2004). Political prints and paper making. *Hand Papermaking, 19*(1), 8–10.

Barron, E., & Gosin, B. (n.d.). Douglas Morse Howell: Papermaking Champion 1906–1994. North American Hand Papermakers. https://www.northamericanhandpapermakers.org/hall-of-champions/douglas-morse-howell.

Bloom, J. M. (2001). *Paper before print: The history of paper in the Islamic world.* Yale University Press.

Boone, C. (2021, December 9). Paper making with older adults and bipolar and related disorders. https://catx63121.wordpress.com/2021/12/09/casey-boone-paper-making-with-older-adults-and-bipolar-and-related-disorders%ef%bf%bc.

Brandstrup, N., Miller, G. M., & Potash, J. S. (2019). Learning from mistakes in adolescent art therapy. In M. Berberian & B. Davis (Eds.), *Art therapy practices for resilient youth: A strengths-based approach to at-promise children and adolescents* (pp. 491–505). Routledge.

Canto, A., McMackin, M., Hayden, S., Jeffery, K., & Osborn, D. (2015). Military veterans: Creative counseling with student veterans. *Journal of Poetry Therapy, 28*(2), 147–163. http://dx.doi.org/10.1080/08893675.2015.1011473.

English Standard Version Bible. (2016). ESV Online. https://www.bible.com/bible/59/ISA.4.ESV.

Fourney, K. (2021). *Applying the healing and transformative nature of papermaking for adolescents with eating disorders.* Unpublished manuscript. Drexel University.

Hinz, L. D. (2009). *Expressive therapies continuum: A framework for using art in therapy.* Routledge.

Hinz, L. D. (2020). *Expressive therapies continuum: A framework for using art in therapy* (2nd ed.). Routledge.

Hunter, D. (1974). *Papermaking: The history and technique of an ancient craft.* Dover Publications.

Kay, L., & Wolf, D. (2017). Artful coalitions: Challenging adverse adolescent experiences. *Art Education, 70*(4), 26–33. https://doi.org/10.1080/00043125.2017.1335542.

King, J. (Ed.). (2016). *Art therapy, trauma, and neuroscience: Theoretical and practical perspectives.* Routledge.

Kramer, E. (1986). The art therapist's third hand: Reflections on art, art therapy, and society at large. *American Journal of Art Therapy, 4,* 71–86.

Leone, L. (Ed.). (2020). *Craft in art therapy: Diverse approaches to the transformative power of craft materials and methods.* Routledge.

Lewis, N. (2009). *I hacky sacked in Iraq.* Combat Paper Press.

Lewis, N. (2012). *Colors of trees we couldn't name.* Combat Paper Press.

Matott, D. (2016, November 30). *Peace paper project: Veteran paper workshop* [Video]. YouTube. https://youtu.be/UU_jiYYMIjo.

Matott, D. L., & Miller, G. M. (2020). Papermaking. In P. Crawford, B. J. Brown, & A. Charise (Eds.), *The Routledge companion to health humanities* (pp. 311–316). Routledge.

McElveen, R. (2007). Using art as therapy. *Vanguard, LIII,* 5. U.S. Department of Veteran Affairs, 18–21. https://www.va.gov/opa/publications/archives/vanguard/07sepoctvg.pdf.

McGrath, J. F. (2022, April). Jesus and the money changers (John 2:13–16). https://www.bibleodyssey.org:443/passages/main-articles/jesus-and-the-moneychangers.

McMackin, M. (2021). Hand papermaking with student veterans. In R. Mims (Ed.), *Art therapy with veterans* (pp. 57–77). Jessica Kingsley Publishers.

McNiff, S. (1998). *Trust the process: An artist's guide to letting go* (1st ed.). Shambhala.

Paige, J. (2021, December 1). *Paper-making for children with learning disorders. Materials, media, and process.* https://catx63121.wordpress.com/2021/12/01/paper-making-for-children-with-learning-disorders

Pennsylvania General Assembly. (2022). Title 18. https://www.legis.state.pa.us/cfdocs/legis/LI/consCheck.cfm?txtType=HTM&ttl=18&div=0&chpt=91.

Perry, B. D. (2009). Examining child maltreatment through a neurodevelopmental lens: Clinical applications of the neurosequential model of therapeutics. *Journal of Loss and Trauma, 14*(4), 240–255.

Philadelphia Police Department. (2022). Crime map & stats. https://www.phillypolice.com/crime-maps-stats.

Rankanen, M. (2014). Clients' positive and negative experiences of experiential art therapy group process. *The Arts in Psychotherapy, 41*(2), 193–204.

Richissin, T. (2004, September). War on Terror "difficult to define." *The Baltimore Sun.* http://seattletimes.nwsource.com/html/nationworld/2002023596_russanal02.html.

Risseeuw, J. (2011). *BOOM! A summary of the paper landmine print project.* Cabbagehead Press.

Rubin, J. (2011). *The art of art therapy: What every art therapist needs to know* (2nd ed.). Routledge.

Stokes, J. (1993). *Thanksgiving address: Greetings to the natural world.* Six Nations Indian Museum.

The Sentencing Project. (2015, November). Americans with criminal records. https://www.sentencingproject.org/wp-content/uploads/2015/11/Americans-with-Criminal-Records-Poverty-and-Opportunity-Profile.pdf.

Trauma. (2020). *Online Etymology Dictionary.* https://www.etymonline.com/search?q=trauma.

U.S. Army Center of Military History. (2021). History of the U.S. army combat artist program. https://history.army.mil/museums/armyArtists/index.html.

U.S. Department of Veterans Affairs. (2021). National Creative Arts Festival. About. https://www.blogs.va.gov/nvspse/national-veterans-creative-arts-festival.

USA Today. (2017). The Wall: Unknown stories, unintended consequences. https://www.usatoday.com/border-wall

Valentino, R. (2013). The combat paper project. *The Iowa Review, 43*(1), 96–100. https://doi.org/10.17077/0021-065X.7307.

Van der Kolk, B. (2014). *The body keeps the score: Brain, mind, and body in the healing of trauma.* Penguin Random House.

Van Lith, T. (2015). Art making as a mental health recovery tool for change and coping. *Art Therapy, 32*(1), 5–12, http://www.doi.org/10.1080/07421656.2015.992826.

Vick, R. (2011). Ethics on exhibit. *Art Therapy, 28*(4), 152–158. http://www.doi.org/10.1080/07421656.2011.622698.

Washington State University. (2021). Undocumented initiatives. https://undocumented.wsu.edu/meet-the-team/yaslin-torres-pe%C3%B1a.

Wolf, D. (2018). Adolescent group art therapy. In C. Haen & N. Boyd (Eds.), *Creative arts-based group therapy with adolescents: Theory and practice* (pp. 69–86). Routledge.

Wolf, D., & King, J. (2021). The juxtaposition of rupture and repair: Exploring trauma and resilience with women on the paths of childbearing, birth, and motherhood. In N. Swan-Foster (Ed.), *Art therapy and childbearing issues* (pp. 21–30). Routledge.

8 Future Thoughts and Directions

Drew Luan Matott and Gretchen M. Miller

Introduction

This chapter explores implications and influences for the future of papermaking as a continued agent for social engagement, art therapy, and a voice for personal growth, change, and recovery. The chapter highlights enduring and emerging practices, applications, and considerations for the next generation of artists, art therapists, activists, and community organizers. Recommendations are also offered to address potential challenges and limitations, ways to strengthen existing methods and approaches, as well as ideas about the future direction of papermaking.

Looking ahead to the next era of papermaking, what could the future bring? To assist us with this inquiry, we invited individuals from the art therapy and papermaking communities to share their thoughts and views. Those who took part included new art therapist Casey Boone, emerging art therapist and student Emma Krueger, art therapist and art therapy educator Dr. Sheila Lorenzo de la Peña, papermaking toolmaker Lee McDonald, and paper artist Patrick Sargent. We were especially curious to explore forward-thinking content about the themes of this book.

Papermaking as Social Engagement

The art and practice of papermaking have experienced an explosion of renewed activity and interest in the U.S., especially as a form of **socially engaged art (S.E.A.)**. With the 2008 invention of McDonald's lightweight and efficient **Oracle Hollander beater** (Paperslurry, 2014) papermaking studios became portable, thereby sharing the experience with communities who may have not been exposed to the process. The old model of bringing community members to a fixed studio was replaced by a more inclusive design that brought papermaking to the streets, community centers, hospitals, and public arenas (Matott, 2008). As a case in point, nearly all the contributors to this book have used or owned one of McDonald's Hollander beaters. This new mode of operation allowed the papermaker to engage in relevant issues where communities reside (P. Sargent, personal communication, 2022).

DOI: 10.4324/9781003216261-12

Civic and Cultural Engagement

With an ever-growing number of activists and artists seeking to use papermaking as S.E.A., using mobile and interactive frameworks encourages expanded collaboration and communal expression. Outreach programs like many shared in this book will continue to have a ripple effect, inspiring new start-ups that address matters impacting communities. In today's uncertain social, political, and environmental climate, the process of papermaking can bring people together to harness their collective power to create change.

While most of this activity has existed within the U.S., over the last few years socially informed papermaking has gained traction internationally. For example, papermaking has been used as a form of reconciliation between warring cultures in the United Kingdom, for the integration and settlement of refugees and migrants in Germany, as a method of expressing repressed cultural identity both in Spain and Poland, as well as for displaced Ukrainian families in Estonia who have been impacted by war (Peace Paper Project, 2022).

Another cross-cultural perspective is papermaking as a form of global recycling. With the burgeoning transnational cannabis industry, there is an opportunity to harness the plant waste from farms for use in the manufacturing of paper. In addition, the textile industry creates an abundance of waste that ends up in landfills worldwide (Benson, 2019). These discarded fibers can be transformed into both **pulp** and paper, becoming a local commodity and income source (Opoku-Asare & Yeboah, 2013).

Hybrid Community Engagement Models

As technologies make it easier for people to interact from the comfort of their homes, it may be beneficial to further adapt how papermaking can be accessed remotely online. Increasing these strategies can allow people to choose how they want to experience the papermaking process. In addition to in-person offerings, imagine how local, regional, and international socially engaged papermaking programs could be conducted in real-time with digital applications such as avatars or virtual reality (Zhong et al., 2020). Bringing materials and concepts out of the private creative setting to create a relationship with participants asynchronously, no matter where they live, can reduce alienation. Virtual programs could also alleviate many physical logistics involved in the papermaking experience. These include, but are not limited to, hauling heavy equipment, buckets full of pulp, soaked **couching** felts and stacks, and securing ample space to manage participant safety and accessibility needs.

Sargent (personal communication, 2022) cautioned however that the hands-on, relational, and tactile attention to the papermaking process, materials, and in-person interactions could lose human connection when delivered through a virtual environment. The use of technology in art therapy has experienced similar concerns (Zubala et al., 2021). Employing technology, just like any tool or application, should consider the needs and goals of the individual, group, or community.

Papermaking as Art Therapy

The momentum gained over the last decade for papermaking as art therapy is positioned to keep growing and flourishing. This book has included several examples of how art therapists, art therapy educators, and art therapy students have used practices in their work, teaching, and studies. The concrete steps of preparing raw and remarkable fibers to transform into pulp offer tangible containment and an emotional framework to release and make meaning of personal experiences, memories, and circumstances attached to the original material. As a form of therapy, the sensory-based process of papermaking invites opportunities for self-soothing and regulation through the physical act of repetition in the here and now. Sheets of paper formed from the reconstituted pulp create an opportunity for repair, renewal, and a shift in awareness (Matott & Miller, 2020).

Non-traditional Practices

The use of unconventional media methods in art therapy has started to grow in diversity and divergence. This is evidenced by current material choices and therapeutic rationale (Leone, 2020), forms of delivery (Partridge, 2021), settings (DelliCarpini, 2020), and attention to social justice issues (Goerdt et al., 2022). Boone (personal communication, 2022) described making paper as a novel art therapy media and process, as Havlena noted in Chapter 5. This creates an increased need for further methods, environment, and population adaptations. Art therapists are encouraged to keep incorporating diversity into how non-traditional media, including hand papermaking, can be implemented (S. Lorenzo de la Peña, personal communication, 2022). Krueger also noted the importance of art therapists therapeutically valuing both the papermaking process *and* product. It is hoped these considerations can motivate further approaches and interventions. This includes individuals, groups, and communities that art therapists work with, in different settings, and additional options for treatment goals, prevention, wellness, and psychosocial functioning.

Trauma Competence and Collaboration

Art therapists can add a trauma-competent voice and clinical awareness when collaborating with community partners on papermaking projects (S. Lorenzo de la Peña, personal communication, 2022). This lens can be valuable when working with vulnerable, marginalized, and at-risk populations, including how papermaking can aid in managing ancestral and generational trauma (E. Krueger, personal communication, 2022). The Peace Paper Project's existing initiative of working in collaboration with art therapists from clinical settings to community art centers as a tool for managing trauma will continue to be important for enhancing, strengthening, and sustaining this endeavor.

Papermaking as Personal Voice

Without reliance on words, papermaking can communicate one's thoughts, feelings, and life experiences, as well as share them with others as a form of validation, remembrance, legacy, or advocacy (Sargent, 2016). As described throughout this book, the methods of expressing personal and community narratives are revealed through conversations with other participants, often while breaking **rag**, and transforming the material, and then later with their friends, family, and neighbors as participants share their experiences of making paper from specific fibers (P. Sargent, personal communication, 2022). Here are some considerations to help strengthen papermaking as a personal voice.

Identity

The metaphor of taking apart, reframing, or repurposing what needs to be or has been altered, discarded, or shifted and creating a new beginning is relevant to the process of self-discovery and transformation (Jacobson-Levy & Miller, 2022). It is vital to welcome an expansion of unique voices and diverse identities to be included, seen, and heard. Papermaking can offer a purposeful way to explore and address identity development, especially in times of transition and change. Particularly noted was how Lesbian, Gay, Bisexual, Transgender, Queer or Questioning (L.G.B.T.Q.+) and other sexual orientation or gender identity communities may find the transformative process of papermaking helpful in exploring and expressing themes associated with one's identity (S. Lorenzo de la Peña, personal communication, 2022). People who are incarcerated would be another population that could re-establish identity and benefit from papermaking (Gussak, 2019). Boone (personal communication, 2022) also advocated further engaging the sensory-based qualities of papermaking with older adults to explore its impacts on identity-related topics about aging, memory, and degenerative health conditions, as well as grief and loss.

Diversity, Equity, and Inclusion

A commitment to diversity, equity, and inclusion (D.E.I.) can also enhance valuing a wide range of narratives and experiences. All ages, populations, and communities can benefit from papermaking. Another reflection includes the narratives and voices that have emerged and have been missing because of forgotten or overlooked forms of making paper, in preference to **Eastern and Western-style** practices. For example, *Cultural Substrates as Paper*, a 2021 North American Hand Papermakers conference panel, explored this topic which included B.I.P.O.C. (Black, Indigenous, and People of Color) quiltmakers, potters, weavers, and book artists. The group of presenters questioned what might arise if handmade paper was viewed "as a vessel for collective memory, as a body, as a site of meaning, or even as an ancestor?" (Blassingame, 2021, para 1). This inquiry has implications not only for existing and emerging papermakers but for practicing and future art therapists to consider in their future work.

Enduring Practices and Emerging Perspectives

Hand papermaking, as well as art therapy, has continually evolved, adapted, and transformed in relation to the material, methods, and applications, while still retaining the core foundations and values of its practice (Levin, 2012; Heller, 1978; Kapitan, 2008). Perpetual growth has helped advance narratives and historical accounts that resonate today. Table 8.1 summarizes the enduring practices and emerging perspectives we have identified. Content also includes feedback noted during our conversations with Boone, Krueger, Lorenzo de la Peña, McDonald, and Sargent (personal communication, 2022).

Table 8.1 Papermaking's enduring practices and emerging perspectives.

Enduring Practices	*Emerging Perspectives*
• Historical, ancestral, and traditional • Traditional use of materials and processes • Adaptability, endurance, flexibility • Sensory-based, somatic process • Contained, concrete, tangible • Transformative process • Destruction/reconstruction, death/birth themes • Communicating, documenting the human experience, storytelling	• Use of technology to enhance and support the papermaking experience • Hybrid D.I.Y. approaches, found and repurposed materials • Collaboration between clinical and community-based practice • Bottom-up brain processing • Increase use of analog, organic, and natural, eco-informed materials • Waste management through upcycling • Dialectical Behavioral Therapy (D.B.T.), strength-based, and post-traumatic growth approaches

Challenges and Limitations

While hand papermaking has experienced renewed interest, there are still numerous obstacles that exist related to sustainability and accessibility.

Sustainability

Throughout its history, papermaking has relied on skilled toolmakers to adapt, design, and build the technology used to render plant matter into paper. The knowledge for tool building is derived from dedicated research and experience in papermaking, woodworking, and metal fabrication (Barrett, 2018). Traditional **paper mills** often had experienced craftspeople who were trained to build and maintain **moulds** and **deckles, presses**, and Hollander beaters.

On the one hand, today anyone who is interested in making paper can visit a website, watch a video, read a book, or attend a workshop or course. The medium itself and learning the process are both much more accessible. However, McDonald states that there is a significant difference between the training of the conventional artisan and a student of the paper arts. The traditional papermaker has spent a lifetime acquiring knowledge and honing their skills, while contemporary paper art students apply basic techniques such as **pulping** and **sheet formation**. Rarely do students learn toolmaking. This discrepancy is of future concern since the number of people who commercially create moulds, deckles, and manufacture Hollander beaters is decreasing. Without a sustained understanding and practice of the fine craft of papermaking and its tools, essential skills may be reduced or possibly lost (L. McDonald, personal communication, 2022).

Accessibility

Despite papermaking being an adaptable medium, Boone, Krueger, and Lorenzo de la Peña all cited accessibility challenges (personal communication, 2022). While information about how to make paper can be easily found, garnering special equipment, such as a Hollander beater, can be difficult, take time, and be expensive. The cost to equip, or the resources available to fund, even the most rudimentary traditional papermaking operation can be challenging or even prohibitive. In addition to expense barriers, papermaking is a labor- and time-intensive process. In preparation for a workshop or session, one can spend several hours planning, processing fibers, managing equipment, setting up, and cleaning. Given the attention needed for these logistics, this can be cumbersome, particularly for a short-term engagement. The process also requires water, therefore special consideration is needed when considering the space. Finally, regardless of whether papermaking is publicly on the streets or privately in a hospital or school, hygienic and safety protocols and any environmental modifications should be assessed and implemented (C. Boone & S. Lorenzo de la Peña, personal communications, 2022). This can include attending to health precautions, acuity, sensory sensitivities, and disability considerations.

Recommendations

We also offer some concrete suggestions for thought. Here are ideas to consider for amplifying and further developing **contemporary papermaking** for social engagement, art therapy, and personal voice.

Education

Learning and teaching through instruction, collaboration, networking, and the exchanging of resources is essential for the continued growth and possibilities of hand papermaking for artists, educators, art therapists, activists, and community organizers:

- **Cultivate the next generation of papermaking toolmakers.** Contemporary paper artists are needed to create fundamental equipment and hardware (L. McDonald, personal communication, 2022). Boone and Lorenzo de la Peña also encouraged art therapists to introduce new methods to streamline how to make paper in a therapeutic setting (personal communication, 2022). Attention to the continued development of unconventional, D.I.Y., inexpensive options can enhance papermaking's reach and application. Perhaps the future of papermaking tools and methods can include collaborations between paper artists, toolmakers, and art therapists.
- **Increase papermaking's visibility as a form of social engagement, art therapy, and personal voice.** Sargent (personal communication, 2022) highlighted the importance of educating others about the value and power of narratives connected to the paper's human element to help sustain engagement and connection. We hope that this book has shed light and awareness on the many benefits of the art and art therapy of papermaking for social action, community, advocacy, emotional expression, and conveying one's story. Equally importantly, we hope that this book encourages and motivates readers to participate in these forms of hand papermaking and share their experiences and stories with others.
- **Develop opportunities for networking, idea, and resource sharing.** There are already many resources on- and offline for learning about how to make paper, where to find tools or equipment, and ways to connect to other papermakers and groups interested in the paper arts. A general web search for "papermaking resources" will lead you to several sites, studios, and links. However, a space dedicated to the sections of this book could be a helpful

resource for those seeking to specifically learn more about these practices and applications, exchange ideas, and connect with other interested individuals. Inspired by this book, we have created http://www.ArtAndArtTherapyOfPapermaking.com to help support these interests.

Scholarship

Education also occurs through engaging in activities of scholarship. This form of knowledge sharing may promote hand papermaking to new audiences, further revealing its advantages and powerful impact:

* Increase the literature available through more published articles, books, and case studies. This additional investigation creates more voices, viewpoints, and diverse ways of working to disseminate (Kapitan et al., 2011). Lorenzo de la Peña noted having scholarly sources could also support grant and funding applications for papermaking (personal communication, 2022). Krueger believed this could further strengthen papermaking's credibility, validity, safety protocols, and best practices (personal communication, 2022).
* Boone (personal communication, 2022) recommended participatory action research (Kapitan et al., 2011) as a valuable approach to learn from qualitative data about papermaking and points of view associated with collected narratives. This also supports more opportunities for ethnographic research. These investigative methods could study art-based insights related to diverse populations, in both clinical and community environments, as well as socially engaged and trauma-informed approaches.

It is difficult to forecast what the future holds or what unexpected encounters will shape our experiences tomorrow. However, using the resources and tools available now empowers us to respond in innovative ways to challenges and opportunities that can influence the future. In closing, we encourage readers to revisit the call for action that we presented at the beginning of the book. We invite you to consider again how the papermaking processes and practices described throughout these pages could be a catalyst for your own creative action. Just like creating handmade paper, the possibilities are full of potential.

References

Barrett, T. D. (2018). *European hand papermaking: Traditions, tools, and techniques.* The Legacy Press.

Benson, E. (2019, January/February). The future of paper. Communication Arts. https://www.commarts.com/columns/the-future-of-paper.

Blassingame, T. (2021). Cultural substrates as paper [Panel]. Primrose Press. https://www.primrosepress.com/nahp-panel1.

DelliCarpini, E. (2020). Breaking bars: Community-based art therapy mural project. *Art Therapy*, *7*(4), 185–193. http://www.doi.org/10.1080/07421656.2020.1824561.

Goerdt, M. N., Gruezo Resurreccion, A. A., Taziyah, B., Johnson, R., Lorenzo de la Peña, S., & Johnson, T. (2022). B.I.P.O.C. art therapists: Antiracism work through the virtual circle. *Art Therapy*, *39*(2), 103–107. http://www.doi.org/10.1080/07421656.2021.2024318.

Gussak, D. (2019). *Art and art therapy with the imprisoned: Re-creating identity*. Routledge.

Heller, J. (1978). *Papermaking*. Watson-Guptill Publications.

Jacobson-Levy, M., & Miller, G. M. (2022). Creative destruction and transformation in art and therapy: Reframing, reforming, reclaiming. *Art Therapy*, *39*(4), 194–202. https://doi.org/10.1080/07421656.2022.2090306.

Kapitan, L. (2008). "Not art therapy": Revisiting the therapeutic studio in the narrative of the profession. *Art Therapy*, *25*(1), 2–3. http:///www.doi.org/10.1080/07421656.2008.10129349.

Kapitan, L., Litell, M., & Torres, A. (2011). Creative art therapy in a community's participatory research and social transformation. *Art Therapy*, *28*(2), 64–73. http://www.doi.org/10.1080/07421656.2011.578238.

Leone. L. (Ed.). (2020). *Craft in art therapy: Diverse approaches to the transformative power of craft materials and methods*. Routledge.

Levin, M. (2012, February). Can a papermaker save civilization? *The New York Times*. https://www.nytimes.com/2012/02/19/magazine/timothy-barrett-papermaker.html.

Matott, D. (2008). Combat paper. Thesis (M.F.A.). Columbia College, Chicago.

Matott, D. L., & Miller, G. M. (2020). Papermaking. In P. Crawford, B. J. Brown, & A. Charise (Eds.), *The Routledge companion to health humanities* (pp. 311–316). Routledge.

Opoku-Asare, N. A., & Yeboah, R. (2013). Hand papermaking with waste fabrics and paper mulberry fibre. *Online International Journal of Arts and Humanities*, *2*(3), 71–82.

Paperslurry. (2014, April). The Oracle Hollander beater – Papermaking equipment by Lee McDonald. https://www.paperslurry.com/2014/08/04/oracle-hollander-beater-papermaking-equipment-lee-scott-mcdonald.

Partridge, E. E. (2021). The pre-research sketchbook: A tool to guide future inquiry. *Art Therapy*, *38*(2), 104–108. http://www/doi.org/10.1080/07421656.2020.1729677.

Peace Paper Project. (2022). Activities. http://www.peacepaperproject.org/activities.html.

Sargent, P. (2016). Echoes of service: Personal narratives and community resilience. George Mason University. https://hdl.handle.net/1920/10498.

Zhong L., Zhou Z., & Xiaopeng, P. (2020). Research on the application of VR technology in the digital inheritance of ancient papermaking technology. *Journal of Physics: Conference Series*, *1453*, 1–5. http://www.doi.org/10.1088/1742-6596/1453/1/012095.

Zubala, A., Kennell, N., & Hackett, S. (2021). Art therapy in the digital world: An integrative review of current practice and future directions. *Frontiers in Psychology*, *12*(595536). http://www.doi.org/10.3389/fpsyg.2021.600070.

Appendix A
Western-style Papermaking Guide

Supplies

Rag material and fiber	Hollander beater
Plastic basin/vat	Mould and deckle
Sizing (optional)	Felt interfacing
Press	Dry box/stack dryer/clothesline

Gathering Rag and Fiber: The first step in making paper is selecting your **rag** or fiber. The key to paper is **cellulose**.

Preparing Rag and Fiber: The second step is to break the weave of the textile and free up the cellulose fibers. Take scissors to the material to remove buttons, zippers, and other non-cellulose material. Then cut into small postage stamp size pieces. **Cooking** the fibers in a caustic solution can help remove grease, dirt, waxes, and detergents. This step is optional, a rinse through hot water will usually suffice.

Pulping with a Hollander Beater: Mix the pieces with water in a **Hollander beater**. This beating systematically hydrates and frees the fibers through intense circulation and pounding to create a **slurry** of **pulp**. At the end of the beating cycle, add a small amount of **sizing**, which helps create less absorbent paper.

Pulling Paper: After the rag is transformed into pulp, the slurry is drained from the Hollander beater into a bucket and scooped into a basin of water, termed a **vat**. The pulp to water ratio determines the thickness of the sheets of paper. If thin sheets are desired, then less pulp is added to the vat and vice versa. **"Charge the vat"** by adding the water and pulp together. Once charged, the **mould** and **deckle** are held together and dipped into the vat. The mould and deckle are **pulled** levelly up from the vat and shaken side to side and front to back. The **shake** is important as it jostles the free fibers into each other to form a **uniform sheet**. **"Hog the vat"** by mixing fibers by hand in between pulling each sheet to evenly distribute the pulp.

Couching: The deckle is then removed from the mould, and the sheet is transferred onto a felted **interface**. A piece of felt is put over the freshly **couched** sheet and this sequence is repeated until the pulp is exhausted and a stack of felts and sheets are formed.

Pressing: Next, push excess water out of the sheets to accelerate **drying** while forcing the cellulose fibers closer together. This allows the sheets to be handled without falling apart. Using a hydraulic, human, or car press are common methods used to **press** paper.

Drying: Paper can be dried with a **dry box**, by hanging from a clothesline, or by laying it out to dry. Once dried, place under a weight until used.

Documentation: A couple of sheets of dried paper can be set aside to document the materials and methods used, including information about the story or content of the fiber.

Appendix B

Do-it-Yourself (D.I.Y.) Papermaking Guide

D.I.Y. Supplies

Paper and cellulose fibers
Wooden stretcher bars or picture frames
Staple gun
Deep plastic bin/vat

Household blender
Window screen
8½ × 11 inch felt sheets for couching
Wooden board or the plastic bin's lid/press

Specialty pulp and inclusions (optional)

Gathering Paper and Cellulose: Basic copy paper creates a smoother, more consistent sheet, while magazine pages and glossy or construction paper tend to blend more irregularly. Pre-made dried **specialty pulps** can be added to help enhance the paper's strength and texture. **Inclusions** such as leaves, flowers, plant fibers, seeds, or spices can also be added during pulping or pulling.

Pulping with a Household Blender: A blender's blades and motor cannot handle fabric. Cut or tear the paper into approximately 1-inch square pieces. Place a couple of handfuls of paper in the blender with enough water to cover the pieces completely. Try not to burn out the blender's motor by loading too much paper. Blend until all large chunks are pulverized. Fill the bin/**vat** with one-third water and pour in the pulp.

Creating a DIY Mould & Deckle: Wooden stretcher bars, commonly used for canvas or picture frames, can make a mould and deckle. Cut a piece of window screening slightly bigger than the size of the mould's frame and staple gun to secure the screen tightly along all sides.

Pulling Paper: Follow the same directions as in Appendix A.

Couching: Transfer the wet paper on the mould face down onto a piece of felt. Use a sponge to absorb excess water from the back before lifting and releasing the paper. For each sheet of newly made paper, place a piece of felt in between and continue stacking.

DIY Pressing: Place a flat surface (such as a wooden board or the bin's plastic lid) on top of the stack of paper. Apply heavy pressure by standing on it or carefully driving a car wheel over the stack.

DIY Drying: Sheets can be dried on a clothesline by hanging each while still on the felt or by removing the paper from the felt to transfer onto a window or flat surface. Once dry, collect the sheets into a stack and keep them flat with a weighted object.

Documentation: Follow the same directions as in Appendix A.

Appendix C
Tools, Equipment, Materials, and Resources

Tools

Arnold Grummer Papermaking Kits	arnoldgrummer.com
Carriage House Paper	carriagehousepaper.com
Harbor Freight Tools	harborfreight.com
Chester Creek Press Mould & Deckle	chestercreekpress.com/moulds.html
Peace Paper Mould & Deckle	peacepaperproject.org/moulds_&_deckles.html

Equipment

David Reina Hollander	davidreinadesigns.com/reina-beater
Oracle Portable Hollander	toolsforpaper.com
Peter Gentenaar Hollander	gentenaar-torley.nl/beater
Valley Beater	dejavulab.com
Hydraulic Press	harborfreight.com/northerntool.com
Papermaking Presses and Drying Box	affordablebindingequipment.com
How to Make a Dry Box	helenhiebertstudio.com/making-a-drying-box

Materials

Interfacing, Felts	carriagehousepaper.com
Pulps in Sheet Form	
Sizing	
Pulps, Fibers, Additives	twinrockerhandmadepaper.com
Specialty Pulps	dickblick.com | arnoldgrummer.com

Resources

Hand Papermaking, Inc.	handpapermaking.org
International Association of Hand Papermakers	iapma.info
North American Hand Papermakers	northamericanhandpapermakers.org

Papermaker's Companion — helenhiebertstudio.com/product-category/books

Papermaking with Garden Plants & Common Weeds — helenhiebertstudio.com/product-category/books

Paperslurry — paperslurry.com

Peace Paper Project Tools & Tutorials — peacepaperproject.org/tools.html

Documentation Sheet

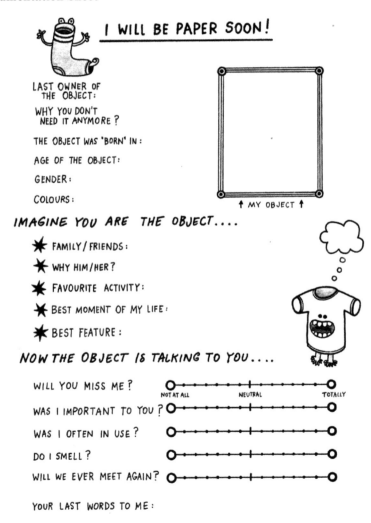

Figure C.1 *I Will Be Paper Soon!* Credit: Julia Münz and Lisa Göppl.

Glossary

Abaca: Banana leaf fiber that is often blended with other papermaking fibers.

Activate/Activating (the paper): To start using or to do something with sheets of paper made. This may be in the form of creative expression through writing, bookmaking, printing, painting, drawing, collaging, or it may be simply gifting the paper to others.

Artist book: A book object that is created as a work of fine art. It often uses physical and conceptual design considerations to dictate an overall experience for the viewer.

Bast fiber: The inner layer of bark from a plant, often long and strong. The most common bast fibers used for papermaking are paper mulberry, flax, hemp, jute, and kenaf.

Blotter: A heavy sheet of unsized paper, most often used to remove moisture from pressed and drying paper.

Broadside: A print that is not bound in a book.

Cellulose: The key component for making paper. Pulp is created as a result of breaking down the cellulose in plant fibers. Papermaking relies on the composition of glucose molecules that naturally fit with water and hydrogen bonding to form the paper's strong structure.

Charge/Charging the vat: The act of adding the pulp to the vat and mixing it in. This action helps evenly distribute the fibers into a homogenized slurry for making sheets of paper by maintaining a consistent pulp-to-water proportion and relative thickness.

Cockling: The wrinkling or rippling of paper due to the fibers' reaction to changing temperature and humidity. This form of buckling can be decreased by managing the environment's humidity and gradually allowing the paper to dry between weighted blotters.

Colophon: A description of authors, location, dates, materials, methods, and techniques used in the creation of a book. It most commonly appears at the end of the book.

Contemporary papermaking: A general term to describe methods of making paper that deviate from traditional papermaking techniques. Pulp painting, pulp printing, socially engaged papermaking, papermaking as art therapy, and interactive and performative papermaking practices are common forms of contemporary papermaking.

Cooking: Cooking the fibers to loosen, clean, and chemically break rag down, to prepare for pulping.

Couch/Couching: Pronounced "cooching." The process of transferring a sheet of paper onto a piece of interfacing material. This sequence is repeated until all the pulp is exhausted and a stack of felts and sheets are formed.

Craftivism: The use of craft and the power of creativity as a voice and to create a better world. A form of art-based activism, this practice is often influenced by social justice, environmentalism, anti-capitalism, the do-it-yourself (D.I.Y.) movement, and third-wave feminism.

Deckle: The chief tool of the papermaker is the mould and deckle. The deckle is the top frame used together with a bottom frame (mould) to give the paper shape when pulling through the pulp to form a sheet of paper.

Deckle box: A mould with a very tall deckle. The tool is clasped together, suspended in water, and pulp is poured on top. Also known as a pour hand mould.

Double couching: A creative sheet forming technique of layering pulps on top of each other by multiple couching.

Double-dipping: A creative sheet-forming technique of merging different pulps directly on the mould by dipping into multiple vats.

Dry box: A tool whereby sheets of pressed papers are layered between blotters and corrugated material and pressure is applied to the stack. Often a fan is used to push air through to expedite drying. Also known as a stack dryer.

Drying: The process of removing water and other wet media from the pulp, allowing for hydrogen bonding of the cellulose to happen. Paper is not fully made until it is dried.

Eastern-style papermaking: A generic term that refers to hand papermaking as it traveled east from its origins in China.

Emulsion: A photosensitive material that can be applied to paper, canvas, or silkscreen to make photographs.

European-style mould and deckle: A two-piece tool made from hardwood consisting of a brass-laid or woven screen.

Fibershed: A local network of farms, mills, textile producers, and consumers in a specific geographical area that grows, sources, and uses fiber from local materials and processing steps to make a product that comes from and within the same region.

Fibrillation: Another term for beating the fiber with a hammer or fine grinding tools in water to create fibers that are hydrated, separated, and refined into a slurry of pulp.

Folio print: A print onto a sheet of paper that is folded in half.

Hog the vat: To mix the pulp by hand after charging. Typically done each time before pulling a new sheet of paper.

Hollander beater: Invented in Holland during the seventeenth century, a machine used to transform old textiles into paper pulp by circulating and pounding material through a bladed roll.

Hydrogen bonding: As paper solidifies and dries, bonding occurs between cellulose and hydrogen molecules.

Inclusions: Materials and/or objects added to the pulps: either in the vat, on the mould, during couching, or even before the pressing. Inclusionary fibers are also added to the pulp for decorative and/or conceptual purposes.

Interface/Interfacing: This refers to the material placed between pieces of freshly couched sheets of paper. This allows for the sheets to be removed, after pressing.

Letterpress: A relief printmaking technique whereby lead type is arranged and printed using a printing press.

Linters: Thick sheets of paper composed of cotton fiber are used as a layer between pressed paper, like a blotter, to aid in the drying process.

Mould: The chief tool of the papermaker is the mould and deckle. The mould is the bottom frame that has a stretched screen over it and is used together with a top frame (deckle) to capture pulp to form a sheet of paper.

Nepalese-style mould: A generic term used to describe a mould with the screen stretched to the frame similar to that of a canvas for painting. Pulps are then poured into the frame and dry directly on the mould.

Oracle (Hollander beater): A portable Hollander beater produced by Lee McDonald. It can be both electric- and human-powered.

Panty Pulping: A program created by Peace Paper Project that used the public pulping of undergarments to generate awareness of sexual and domestic violence.

Papermaker tears: The impressions of water droplets on a freshly formed and/or couched sheet of paper.

Paper mill: An enclosed location that is dedicated to the manufacturing of paper.

Pellon®: Often used to describe interfacing, a material that a freshly formed wet sheet of paper is couched on. Papermakers use many materials as interfacing, the most common is a non-fusible polyester, of which Pellon is one brand.

Post: Refers to the layers of interfacing and couched sheets. Usually, the post is capped at the bottom and top with a piece of wood, allowing for equal distribution of pressure during the pressing.

Press/Pressed/Pressing: Crucial to making paper, it pushes the water out of the sheets to quicken the drying process while forcing the cellulose fibers closer together. This process increases hydrogen bonding, allowing the sheets to be handled. Pressing paper can be done with a hydraulic press or simply by standing on the paper stack (human press) or by driving the weight of a car over the stack (car press).

Pull/Pulled/Pulling: The action of removing a combined mould and deckle from a slurry of pulp.

Pulp/Pulped/Pulping: The composition of plant-based material that has been freed from its textile or plant structure and suspended in water. Synonymous with slurry. Pulping is the act of using water and force to separate cellulose-based textiles or raw plants into usable material for papermaking.

Pulp chips: Individually packaged, sterile, and dehydrated pulp that can be reconstituted with distilled water for making paper. This application is particularly important for creating a hygienic papermaking process in medical settings.

Pulp painting: A creative sheet forming application that relies on layering pulps, such as pulp printing, double couching, double dipping, and using pulp as a writing and/or drawing media.

Pulp printing: A wet printmaking process that uses finely beaten pulp fibers to stencil print onto couched sheets of paper. Commonly done by disbursing pigmented pulp through a spray bottle with a coarse silkscreen stencil.

Rag: A textile that is awaiting to be processed into pulp. "Breaking rag" is a term used when engaging in the steps of transforming textiles into paper pulp: i.e., cutting, tearing, cooking, and beating.

Reina (Hollander beater):   A line of stainless-steel Hollander beaters manufactured by David Reina.

Restraint drying: The process of drying paper in a way that restricts shrinkage and warping.

Shake/Shaking: The act of gently but firmly jostling the mould and deckle after it is pulled from the vat. This action helps intermingle the pulp fibers to create a smooth, non-lumpy surface for the finished paper.

Sheet formation: The process of making a sheet of paper. There are two general methods of sheet-forming: pulling and pouring.

Sizing: A non-cellulose material that is added to the pulp and/or finished paper and used to slow the absorption of wet media. There are two primary methods of sizing: external and internal. External sizing (also known as surface sizing) uses a gelatin bath or rice/wheat flour paste can be brushed onto the outside of the paper to coat it. Internal sizing is added at the end of the beating to get in between the plant fibers.

Slurry: Beaten fiber suspended in any amount of water. Synonymous with pulp.

Socially engaged art (S.E.A.):   The creation, use, and/or display of art to educate, inform and/or create a dialogue about topics focused on community, society, collaboration, and social action.

Specialty pulps: Acid-free, pre-shredded, and blender-friendly dried pulp that adds softness and strength to handmade paper. Specialty pulps are often available in cotton, denim, wool, corn husk, and Kona fiber to use exclusively or in combination with existing pulp.

Uniform sheet: A sheet of paper that has been formed evenly, so it does not have uneven sides or lumpy or broken formation.

Valley (Hollander beater):   Manufactured by Valley Iron Works, this Hollander beater was originally designed as a lab machine for industrial paper mills to conduct small test loads. It has recently been re-appropriated by hand papermakers.

Vat: A basin that is partially filled with water and pulp.

Western-style papermaking: A general term referring to the history and development of papermaking techniques as they traveled westward from their origins in China through the Middle East, Europe, and North America.

Index

For Product Safety Concerns and Information please contact our EU
representative GPSR@taylorandfrancis.com
Taylor & Francis Verlag GmbH, Kaufingerstraße 24, 80331 München, Germany